Healthy and Fit
with Tai Chi

Healthy and Fit with Tai Chi

PERFECT YOUR POSTURE, BALANCE AND BREATHING

Sifu Peter Newton

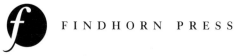

FINDHORN PRESS

Published in 2015 by Findhorn Press, Scotland

ISBN 978-1-84409-656-5

Edited by Jacqui Lewis
Illustrations by Jeff Cushing
Cover design by Richard Crookes
Interior design by Damian Keenan
Printed & bound in the EU

Published by

Findhorn Press

117-121 High Street,

Forres IV36 1AB,

Scotland, UK

t +44 (0)1309 690582

f +44 (0)131 777 2711

e info@findhornpress.com

www.findhornpress.com

Contents

Foreword
by
Dr Yang, Jwing-Ming

I first met Peter Newton more than ten years ago at one of my seminars in England. We continued to cross paths several times after our first meeting. I became impressed with his enthusiasm for learning, practising and teaching; and from his new book I can see just how much progress he has made over the last decade.

Peter's book provides readers with a wealth of information in Tai Chi and Qigong. Whether you are looking to improve your health, maintain your body or just calm your mind, this book will provide you with a path to get there. I am happy to see teachers like Peter openly share their knowledge and experiences with others. Knowledge should be constantly shared, and with cooperation and friendship. Only then will we be able to achieve a higher spiritual level in the world and a better state of overall being.

As is traditionally known in China, Tai Chi and Qigong are two of the most common, most effective methods for healing, sickness prevention and physical-body maintenance. Nowadays, countless documents have been translated, researched and proven to show the benefits of these practices. Not only do they bring you a calmer and more confident state of mind, they also rebuild your body's balance, endurance, centre and rooting. I hope to see more publications about Tai Chi and Qigong in the future. We all have the power within ourselves to heal, strengthen and change lives. Every person needs to know about it.

— *DR YANG, JWING-MING*
Director, YMAA CA Retreat Center
June 14, 2014

Preface

There is a traditional saying in China: *"It is easier to climb a mountain and catch a tiger than ask for help."* This relates to the many people who find it difficult to seek advice over something that may be simple to answer. But for the sake of seeking advice, lives could be saved and quality of life improved. I therefore decided to dedicate this book to "Self-Help" and "Self-Healing", and by doing so create an additional weapon in the fight against ill-health.

Ever since I can remember I have had a strong interest in health and especially healing. As a child I would search the newspapers and magazines for the "Dear Doctor" pages, soaking up all the advice being administered to a wanting readership by the medical experts. So by the time I was in my early twenties I was beginning to think I would train to become a paramedic, because of the "hands-on" immediate effect they have in helping people. Running in parallel with this was a yearning to explore my artistic nature, which probably explains why in the end I refrained from doing this training. I felt there was something else I needed to find, that was more suited to me; but had no idea what that would be until one day in the summer of 1979 when I switched my television on. What appeared was an old Chinese gentleman, who must have been in his nineties; he walked on to my TV screen looking sprightly and performed a series of choreographed postures with such grace, poise and dexterity that it immediately captured my attention. Although I had no clue then as to the long-term effect that what the Chinese gentleman was demonstrating would have on my life, somehow I knew that it was a special moment. This was the first time I had felt the force of what are known as "Ancient Chinese Power Postures", beaming out from the screen, filling the room like a ray of sunlight. A Tai Chi master had just appeared on my radar and, suitably inspired, I commenced my search for a teacher.

It took me six months to find one, in the form of a Chinese Gung Fu martial arts school less than an hour's drive from my home, where I was taught Wing

Chun and Tai Chi. The Wing Chun did not suit my six-foot-four-inch frame, but I persevered, because they would only teach me the Tai Chi after I'd had Wing Chun training. As soon as I started training in Tai Chi, I realized it fitted me like a warm glove; so not only had it "looked" right for me that first time I saw it, it "felt" right for me the first time I tried it.

Since then, I have had the honour of training with three great Tai Chi and Qigong masters: Chu King Hung, Michael Tse and Dr Yang, Jwing-Ming, who collectively have gifted me the insights, skills and knowledge to be able to share with you these profound health-rejuvenating messages from ancient China.

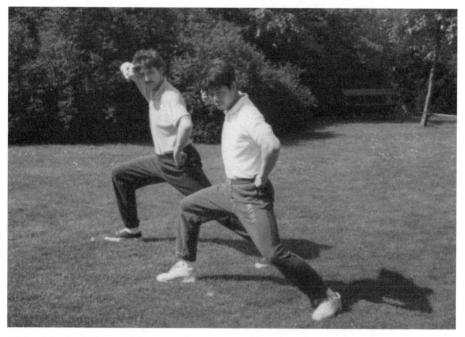

Michael Tse (and the author)

My understanding of the human body's physiology and structure comes not just from the exceptional Tai Chi and Qigong training I have received from the masters, but also derives from my early work background. Throughout the 1970s I worked as a qualified plumbing and heating engineer, which has strangely (or maybe not so strangely) added to my understanding of the fluid circuitry of the human body's physiology. The central-heating pump: the heart; the boiler = Dan Tien (central field of heating energy, located in the core of the abdomen); the pipes = blood vessels; the electrical circuit and thermostatic controls

= central nervous and glandular systems; and the radiators = organs and skin tissue. I knew from installing, commissioning and maintaining these systems that certain rules had to be applied, otherwise the boiler and the pump would face excessive wear and tear and not achieve their life expectancy. The best plumbing and heating engineers, when commissioning a system, would know it was balanced and working efficiently just by looking, listening, feeling and even smelling. All the things that a Traditional Chinese Medicine doctor does when diagnosing a patient.

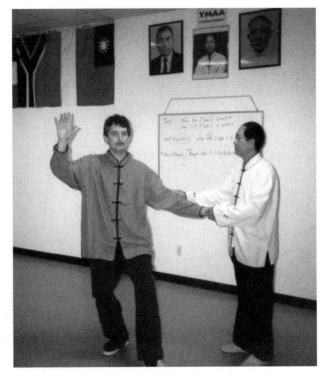

Master Dr Yang, Jwing-Ming (and the author)

My work in construction management throughout the 1980s and into the 1990s also contributed to my understanding of human structures. This job required me to have intimate knowledge of building and engineering structures: foundation and floor slabs = feet; walls, columns and stanchions = skeletal frame, and the roof = the head. I discovered that gravity works on building structures in exactly the same way as on the human body. For there to be structural integrity, gravitational force must remain in the centre of the physical joints and frame.

A final point to mention on structures is that, through the martial aspects of Tai Chi Chuan, my teachers taught me the importance of accuracy of structure in the martial postures and applications of the same – this has given me a much deeper understanding of body engineering than I would have acquired if I had only concentrated on the health and healing aspects of this art/science.

In my first two books *Tai Chi and Qigong: The Ultimate Beginner's Guide* and *The Middle Path of Tai Chi*, I attempted to provide readers with a practical introduction. In this book, however, I decided to focus purely on how to help people apply this knowledge for everyday healthy living. Generally, I cover the health benefits and curative effects of good posture, correctness of body-mechanics in motion and how to realize optimum performance in neurological, respiratory, cardiovascular, lymphatic and general organ functions. This is not intended to be a medical scientific-reference journal: on the contrary, it is simply a practical and fascinating guide to the ancient Chinese way of rectifying and enhancing health with movement and posture at its core.

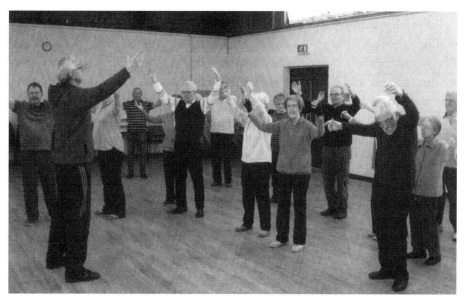

The author working with a group of Parkinson's patients

For many years, I have recognized that the body-shapes performed in Tai Chi Chuan and Qigong are not just mechanics for general health and self-defence. I noticed early on that they projected a force, a kind of radiant energy that eventually I could even detect emanating from a still photograph. This was the power within the postures and for the last two decades I have been developing, evaluating and applying this power, both in helping people with serious medical conditions and in showing the more able-bodied how to utilize this power for general health and longevity. This work and its ongoing results, which I share with you throughout the book, are enlightening, rewarding and humbling.

In my book *The Middle Path of Tai Chi*, I introduced the "real" hidden meaning of Tai Chi Chuan and Qigong. Now I progress this educational journey by showing and describing how the Middle Path is in fact the source and conduit for this power. To complement the illustrations and commentary, I have strategically placed a variety of selective Chinese quotations, proverbs and my own constructed poetic verses; they collectively shed light on this innate, natural human healing power (Ren Qi).

"The best doctor cures people before they become ill."
— CHINESE PROVERB

So who is this book written for? It is for everyone who has an interest in their health and general well-being and, with the global scientific world's interest in Tai Chi and Qigong now at unprecedented levels, *now* is the time. In over thirty-four years of involvement in these amazing arts, I have never seen so many funded research projects being carried out by reputable scientific institutions, which is why I have included a chapter dedicated to their latest findings.

"How can an unhealthy doctor make someone healthy?"
— CHINESE PROVERB

The book has been structured to make it easy for someone new to these arts to assimilate this important knowledge; each chapter is laid out as an informative lecture with a Q&A session at the end. The questions chosen are selected from those that I have been (and continue to be) asked by my enthusiastic and inquisitive new students.

A Dedication

Finally, I would like to dedicate this book to Ian Begbie, my late teaching colleague and friend. After an immense battle with not one, but two life-threatening illnesses, Ian proved that nature's self-healing power can extend life far beyond the expectations of the medical experts. Ian was a trained senior nurse specializing in orthopaedics and, although I was his teacher, *he* taught *me* much about the structural body and human health generally. It helped make me the teacher I am today. Although Ian did finally succumb (years beyond when he was expected to), he showed that by utilizing the force that had been placed in him by the Dao, she (the Dao, that is) was happy to allow him to spend more time with his family and friends before finally calling his name.

Once again I am with great pride reintroducing the ancients' "Way" to a healthy life.

Peter Newton

1

Introduction to Self-Healing Power

A force for all, a force on call,
A force that cannot be forced.
— PTN

The first thing to explain is the concept of a self-healing power. Western medicine has only recently acknowledged that poor posture correlates to poor health. In regards to this, medical professionals are now advising their patients on the benefits of good posture; something that in Asia has always been part of the fabric of their holistic approach to medicine. Since ancient times Asian doctors have understood that not only does poor posture create specific poor health conditions, but good posture will equally act to create uniquely beneficial healing conditions.

Body language also plays its part as it manifests through postures and expressions, which in themselves tell a tale to the observer about the state of health, mind and spirit of the individual. The self-healing potential of an individual can also depend on other factors such as:

AGE – Older people (fifty and older) take longer to heal than younger people.

ATTITUDE – A person who is willing to accept healing with an open mind and no fixed expectations will obtain better results than those who show reluctance to do the same.

SHAPE/SIZE – Tall, short, slim, fat, heavy muscular, light muscular, frail and strong: a typical room will contain people answering to all these descriptions, who because of their specific shapes/sizes will assimilate healing in differing ways.

LIFESTYLE – The way an individual conducts his or her life: for example, living in the fast lane or being sedentary will both have a direct impact on the body's self-healing potential.

DIET – Those who consume excessively or under-consume, even if it is healthy food, will weaken their bodies sufficiently to hinder natural healing.

PERSONAL HABITS – Smoking, drinking, drug addiction and excessive or obsessive behaviour all have a negative effect.

"We are what we repeatedly do."
 — *ARISTOTLE*

GENETIC MAKE-UP – This is one area in which self-healing potential can confidently be said to vary immensely; we are all as unique as our thumbprints and some families are known to have the "longevity genes" that protect them all from the ravages of life, while others are plagued by a weakness in their genes that can be passed on from generation to generation. In addition, if a person has a congenital underlying condition, this too will influence their rate of healing potential.

It is against this backdrop that I decided to first isolate and explain "self-healing power" as part of the rich tapestry of measures that create a Middle Path healthy life. In this regard, I decided to select and promote the most common postures seen across the arts of Tai Chi and Qigong, such as Mountain Posture, Earth Posture, Heaven Posture and Hold the Centre Posture (see Chapter 5). Separated out from their usual choreographed patterns within the practices, they have proven that even alone they are health-enhancing postures that can combat a number of adverse health conditions. They operate in three distinct ways:

- **Physically** – how the shapes regulate the human body structure and physiological functions.

- **Mentally** – positively affecting the mental health of an individual.

- **Spiritually** – influencing what the ancient Chinese call the Shen (Living Spirit) of the human body.

The Root of Healthy Living

The Daoist (nature's way) arts of Tai Chi Chuan (TCC) and Qigong jointly form the root source of my "knowledge", so below I will explain their meaning and how they uniquely contribute to the Middle Path method (see Chapter 3). This methodology derives from Tai Chi's martial arts postures (in stillness and in motion), the mechanics of Qin Na (the martial engineered controlling of the body's joints), associated physical conditioning exercises, Shen (Living Spirit) training and martial breathing skills. Add this to Qigong's therapeutic exercises, massage techniques, breathing therapy (Huxi) and body-mechanics and collectively they create skills that are extremely effective in combating and preventing human health conditions.

Tai Chi Chuan

The ancient art of Tai Chi Chuan is often portrayed as the beautiful and graceful dance-like exercise elderly Chinese people do in the park in the mornings and is seen as "nice to watch, but complicated to do" by many Westerners. So when I am asked "What is Tai Chi, what will it do for me and how often should I practise?" I explain as follows:

> In the Western world we are obsessed with abbreviation and have therefore shortened the name to Tai Chi. By doing this, however, we are missing out the most important message in its title: the essence and meaning of "Chuan". Tai Chi = Grand Ultimate, and Chuan = Fist or Boxing, so when they are combined you have the art of Grand Ultimate Fist/Boxing. If we isolate the word Chuan, it is in fact how the ancient Chinese were trying to portray what we understand as "Force". So now we have "The Grand Ultimate Force", which is … nature. The ancient Chinese symbol of the twin forces of nature (the dynamic forces of Yin and Yang that drive the universe) is known as the Tai Chi T'u (Grand Ultimate Symbol) as shown on the following page.

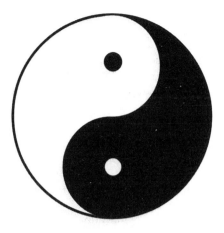

FIGURE 1: Tai Chi T'u

Nothing can compare to these awesome forces at work; they are able to simultaneously create chaos, order and balance throughout the universe. The ancients, however, identified that there was a singular force behind the Yin and the Yang, which they called "The One". Another name for it is "The Dao", which translates as "The Way of Nature". It is made up of the creative Yang and the destructive Yin, the twin opposing and harmonizing forces that manifest in all things. It has been described by the great twentieth-century Tai Chi master Chen Man-Ching as below:

"Its surface is expansive, its centre is cohesive."
— *CHEN MAN-CHING*

So what is Tai Chi Chuan? It is the art of developing naturalness in stillness and motion. What will it do for me? It will return you to nature. And when asked "How often should I practise these postures and movements?" my stock answer is: "How often do you wish to become natural – once a day or twice a week?"

The shapes that the ancient Tai Chi Chuan masters sculpted out of the human body are intended to reflect the Tai Chi symbol.

This forms the bedrock of self-healing power: shapes that carry spirit, strength and subliminal messages to those who observe them. In this context it is correct to state:

"Shapes have meaning."
— *PTN*

Qigong

As Tai Chi Chuan is known for its martial arts origins, Qigong is equally known for its health-promoting benefits. The name means "Energy Skill or Exercise" and it is designed to stimulate and regulate the "Energy Body" (Jinglo). It is said that if the Jinglo is free from stagnation and circulates naturally, the body, mind and spirit all benefit. The shapes the body makes when practising Qigong connect us to the ancient masters who have respectfully nurtured this amazing health science throughout its evolution, a period spanning some 5,000 years. Long before TCC became established, the two major strands of Qigong, Medical and Spiritual, were adopted by the Chinese to enhance their physical and spiritual health. In general, they were practised as individual exercises: for example Qigong for the back, or the neck, or for the whole body (this would be a choreographed combination of movements known as a Qigong Set or Form).

Since the birth of the art of TCC during the Chinese Song Dynasty, in around AD 1200, Qigong has generally been regarded as the engine and TCC the vehicle. Together, they offer us in these hectic modern times an incredibly rich source of scientific research material.

Medical Tai Chi and Qigong

When you delve deeper into these arts you will find the more focused therapeutic interpretation, which has for thousands of years been attached to the range of treatments offered within Chinese Traditional Medicine. To see the purer medical methods in practice you would have to visit the traditional medicine hospitals in China, who have adopted it as part of their holistic approach to natural healing and treatment.

So what is meant by Medical Tai Chi and Qigong? The word "Medi" means "Middle", and that is what TCC and Qigong are designed to do – to find the Middle Path of mind, body and spirit. This is achieved through the way they produce homeostasis, or balance, by encouraging the body to become fully integrated and coordinated. It is only in recent times that TCC has been viewed as medical, as Qigong was historically considered the one and only discipline for this. It all changed in the 1950s when a Hong Kong based Tai Chi and Qigong master combined the two, creating Tai Chi Qigong. Nowadays, this unique combination of Tai Chi healing power postures and medical Qigong postures is practised worldwide and through regular practice the following benefits will manifest:

- Enhancement of circulation.
- Stimulation of acupuncture meridians.

- Respiration and body-motion united in harmony.
- Physical balance while in motion.
- Lymphatic-fluid propulsion.
- Core centring and coordination.
- Gravitationally centring all structural joints of the body.
- Rotation and flexion of joints along natural paths.
- A mind that is clearer and more focused.

The Five Regulators of Healing (Wu Tiao)

The sequence of guiding a person back to the self-healing Middle Path is made up of the "Five Regulators"; below I list the sequence in order. Those highlighted in bold are the primary regulators, with "Respiration" and "Qi" being secondary.

Body

Respiration

Mind

Qi

Spirit

The Western way to collectively describe complementary therapies always places them in the order Mind, Body and Spirit. In practice, however, as can be seen above, they should be approached in the order of Body, Mind and Spirit:

- A restructured and regulated **Body** creates natural Respiration.

- A regulated **Mind** inside a regulated body creates healthy Qi.

- A regulated body and mind reinforces the **Spirit** home.

Philosophy of Health and Healing

"Anything great is long in making."
— LAO-TSU

This relates to the general rule of healing: "What has taken many years to damage will equally take many years to remedy." This does not mean, however, that the benefits of practice will take years to manifest: to the contrary, a person's quality of life will be enhanced from the first step.

"Mankind cannot avoid death and disease."
— WEN ZHUANG

Some people can manifest self-destructive tendencies, but even those who live a healthy, trouble-free Middle Path life will eventually succumb to the all-powerful force of nature the Chinese call "The Dao".

"Eat less, taste more."
— ANCIENT CHINESE SAYING

What obviously applies to our modern-day obsession with food can also relate to other facets of life. For example, if you crave anything too much, when you finally get your wish you may well devour it and not savour it. The warning here is to steer away from excessive yearning and learn to appreciate what you have already got.

"No medicine is as good as a 'Middling Doctor'."
— ANCIENT CHINESE MAXIM

What (I hear you say) is a middling doctor? It is a doctor who does not stand out, who has quietly progressed through his or her training and practice. Who does not make waves, is humble and, because of who they are, sees life from all angles. A person who is open to new ideas and calls upon life's accumulated experience to reinforce theoretical knowledge when treating his or her flock. It is a doctor who walks the "Middle Way" and by doing so truly listens to their patients.

The Power at the Source

Having looked at the source, it is now time to turn to the power of self-healing, which can be split into three different categories: Qi, Ching and Shen, also known as the "Three Treasures".

Qi

This is the life force of the universe that pervades all living matter. It is, therefore, that which gives all living things life. Healthy Qi also manifests to nourish and strengthen the human body through the ingestion of healthy food, drink and air, which collectively materialize as the body's "Vital Energy". For a body to function effectively and healthily, it must have the required levels of Qi. The desired level is set not by ourselves, but by allowing the Dao to function as it wishes within our bodies and minds (living according to nature's laws), which explains the Chinese saying:

"The Dao is without and the Dao is within."

The ancient Chinese discovered that when a human opens the body and mind to the "External Dao", "the Dao within" strengthens and functions optimally. How you physically achieve this is covered later on; however, it is worth pointing out that you are not subject to an external Dao and a second, internal Dao. There is only "One" and according to Lao-tsu, the original famous Daoist master who lived around 500 BC, *"The 'One' (Dao) is 'Mysterious' and 'Inexplicable'."*

How do you train a bird to fly?
How do you tell the best to try?
How does a hawk know how to prey?
And how do you teach a child to play?
How does a snowflake form in the sky?
Ask the Dao to tell you why.

— PTN

Ching

This is what the ancients call the "Original Essence". It is the seed of human life that originally came from our parents. It is linked to the immune system and is stored in the kidneys to protect newborn babies during their first few months of life, until they start to generate their own Ching.

It is important to nurture this Original Essence throughout one's life. This can be achieved by regulating sexual emissions: the "Coarse Qi", as Ching is also called, acts like a fuel-source to the "Vital Qi", which is our life force; when it is depleted, the life force weakens. The ancient Daoists devised an internal breath-driven, meditative alchemic process to transmute Coarse Qi into "Refined Qi". This method is reliant on the adept having first conserved his or her Ching (body fluids generated by the sexual organs), by refraining from sexual ejaculation during intercourse and directing its energy instead up and around the "Small Heavenly Cycle" (see Chapter 3).

Shen

In the context of this book "Shen" is the "Living Spirit" that radiates out from a body that has excellent posture and a positive mind. Shen is visible (and can also be sensed) even when the body is still, radiating out like a light from the core. It manifests in a body in motion as grace, strength and power and according to the ancient teachings: *"Directs the Qi to move the body through a subtle union between the 'Eyes', that focus where to move to and the 'Mind', that motivates the action."*

An example of how the Shen can be visible and is timeless is seen in the incredible postures of the ancient Chinese Terracotta Army. It is said that the figures are based on actual warriors and were buried alongside Emperor Qin Shi Huang Di during the period 210–209 BC. Huang Di was responsible for unifying all the independent warring states into what we now recognize as China. So powerful is the warriors' "Shen Warrior Living Spirit" that it still shines through their inanimate clay bodies to this day. I even sensed its presence (although diffused) in a poor-quality replica of one of the warriors I recently saw in a local garden centre.

> *Shen affects mood and mood affects Shen.*
> — *PTN*

Shen is bolstered and intimately fed by Qi and Qi is bolstered and intimately fed by Ching – this is the natural order of things.

> *Shen is not threatening,*
> *Shen holds no fear,*
> *Shen is timeless and*
> *Shen is clear.*

Shen is subservient,
Shen is true,
Shen is your spirit and
Shen therefore, is you.
— *P T N*

Other Treasures

Although it is generally accepted that Qi, Ching and Shen are *the* Three Treasures, there are other treasures:

Strength relies on the singularity
Of body, mind and spirit.
The coming together of all three
To forge a union of one.
— *P T N*

The great Daoist sage Ko Hung (AD 200–300 approx) refers to a different three in the following reflection on his blissful existence as a recluse, away from society:

"Here I am in the company of my three friends: the moon, my shadow and peace."

This revered sage is sharing his love of the kinship he has with nature and it is this deceptively simple view that best illustrates the most important message when explaining the power behind self-healing. For Ko Hung, contentment came through solitude in nature's cathedral, where he found true peace.

Questions and Answers

I have never experienced this 'Power', so how can I find it?

You say you have not experienced this power, but I would suggest that you have – on numerous occasions. The body's inner healing power or life force (Qi) has been with you since you were born. For example: if you have ever cut or grazed your skin, your healing power was activated the moment you received the wound. Nature (the Dao) simply stepped in and healed the tissues without you needing to do a thing. Another quick way of sensing your own Qi is to imagine you are holding a football in your hands, slightly in front of your navel. Lift your chest slightly and breathe in and you should notice the hands drift naturally apart. Now lower your chest and breathe out and your hands should drift back in as if shrinking the ball. Just do this for two minutes and you will feel your own life force.

What effect would excessive sexual activity have on a person's health?

It all depends on their age. For example, for someone in their early twenties the draining of the Ching caused by excessive sexual emissions would have less of an impact on their immune system (Guardian Qi) than for someone in their fifties. The younger person, however, would still notice that they were catching more colds and viruses than someone else of the same age who was less promiscuous. The difference between a twenty-year-old and a fifty-year-old is that the younger person would recover far quicker than the fifty-year-old, who also runs the risk of long-term kidney and bladder damage (this usually manifests as backache and urinary infections respectively).

Is Qi visible?

The short answer is … yes, even to the untrained eye. We are able to see whether someone is tired or energized by their general appearance. Qi can be seen as: colourful complexion, brightness of the eyes, animated as opposed to lank hair and posture that is upright, strong and purposeful in motion.

The ancient Chinese trained in another level of viewing Qi, which resulted from the regular stimulation of the "Third Eye", otherwise known as the Yintang acupuncture point, located mid-forehead. Also called the seat of the sixth sense or the "Sky Eye", this is where our psychic potential dwells and works in conjunction with the physical eyes to "see" the aura-linked Guardian Qi of a person.

What is the difference between Shen and ghost Spirit?

The Chinese call ghosts "Trapped Spirits", also "Hungry Ghosts"; they are in fact Living Spirits (Shen) that through some strong yearning or drama have become earthbound. Before whatever trauma afflicted them they had the same Shen as you or I. However, when they died, their once natural and healthy Shen transformed into a state of extreme Yang (maligned), or extreme Yin (emotional but usually benign). Thus the term "Hungry Ghosts", meaning they hunger for something so powerfully they could not have when alive that it traps and transforms their Shen, which is now unable to be at rest.

Can Qi be harmful?

Only if you decide to force Qi with overindulgence and impatience, when it will create excessive Yang Qi in the body. This disrupts your natural balance and can make you angry, hyperactive and restless. Similarly, too much concentration on the internal aspects, such as too much meditation, can create excessive Yin Qi, weakening body, mind and spirit. The ideal balance is to train in such a way that you develop "stillness in action" (see Chapter 8), which is inwardly quiet and calm, while outwardly animated with good posture.

2

Tai Chi and
Qigong Classics –
The Root to Self-Healing

How minuscule mere words can be
To describe this gift of ages.
Sent down from misty mountains
Bestowed on man by sages.

— *PTN*

This will be the chapter all others refer to, for here lies the root of self-healing. The Classics are the documented records of the ancient Tai Chi and Qigong masters who describe how to apply the postures and shapes within the body to maximize the flowing and healing Qi potential. The Tai Chi Classics have been written and rewritten by many scribes over the centuries and all without exception start at the head and work their way progressively down the body. Conversely, the Qigong Classics commence at the feet and work their way progressively upwards, covering some key points the Tai Chi Classics do not mention. Together however, they provide a comprehensive and enlightening insight into nature's recommended shapes and structures for the human frame.

"Straightening his belly (abdomen), pulling up his back
(lifting the crown), he achieves proper alignment."
— *I CHING*

As you can see from this gem plucked from the pages of the revered *I Ching*, or *Book of Changes* (circa 1000 BC), the ancient Chinese were aware of "Classic Healthy Posture".

The Tai Chi Classics

The original Classics have been attributed to the great warrior monk and sage Chang San Feng (AD 1200–1400), who on Wudang Mountain in the southern region of Hubei Province devised the art of Tai Chi Chuan. In support of his embryonic art he is said to have written an instruction manual listing the essential components in the creation of a Tai Chi body. And what is a "Tai Chi body"? It is a body that moves in an optimal way, perfectly tuned in to the forces of gravity and universal energy (Qi), which influences everything in the universe (Dao). A maxim often quoted in Tai Chi schools describes what the Tai Chi Classics will do for a person who adheres to their guidance:

> *"Tai Chi will give you the strength of a lumberjack, the suppleness and pliability of a child and the mind of a sage."*

Chang San Feng's original Classics have gone on to be adopted and adapted, initially by the disciples and followers of Wudang Tai Chi Chuan School and thereafter by the five major families of Tai Chi Chuan: Chen, Yang, Wu, Woo and Sun. Each of these schools applies their own interpretation of the Classics and as such they may vary slightly in number and description, depending on where you study and what you read. I decided to generally keep to the Yang School Classics, because that is what most of my training drew on. In addition, there are those Classics that plainly deal only with martial technique, which is not covered in this book, unless they offer an insight into the human posture.

There are five External Classics, which deal with the physical structuring of the body and are intended to iron out the kinks that cause blockages. Then there are the five Internal Classics, intended to enhance the flow of healthy Qi and strengthen the Living Spirit (Shen). The External create the physical conditions for healthy circulation, while the Internal Classics fuel that circulation. Here, I will provide details of the External Classics only, but where appropriate will make reference to the Internal.

I have in the past seen the Classics being misunderstood and misread; particularly, students sometimes tend to hold their bodies stiff in an attempt to achieve the described postures and shapes. The Classics are only a snapshot of what should be a "Living Form" (see Chapter 6); that is, a body in motion, guided by the positions described but not held stiffly in them.

Note: To help apply the Classics, these are the key words for correctness of Tai Chi practice: Smooth, Rounded, Soft, Coordinated, Integrated, Opening, Closing, Natural Lightness, Natural Heaviness and Seamless. You should also follow the notes provided underneath.

1. **Lift the crown of the head as if suspended from a cloud.**
   To suspend the head as described in this maxim, it is important first to locate the "Baihui" (Hundred Convergences) crown point cavity (see Figure 11, page 61). To lift and centre the head correctly, you can visualize a strand of hair being attached to and gently pulled upwards by a string, which at its other end is connected to a cloud. This cloud is elevating the string, but in such a gentle way that the head appears to be floating. The first noticeable benefit will be sensed throughout the whole body: everything below the crown will physically straighten out. This creates "Central Equilibrium" in the skeletal structure, encouraging lightness and agility in the feet and body generally (see Figure 2).

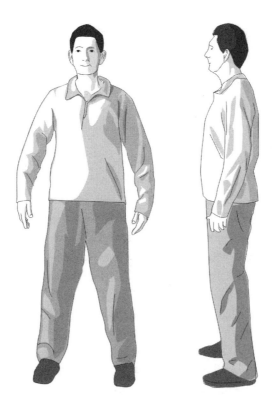

FIGURE 2: The Structure Aligned

The reason for this improvement is due to the formidable force of gravity "finding its home" in the centre of the joints. In addition, the breathing function will instantly operate more efficiently as the lungs and diaphragm are no longer oppressed by poor posture.

"The ancients kept their bodies united with their souls."
— *CH'I PO IN THE NEI CHING*

NOTES

- When lifting up the head from the Baihui (Crown Point), avoid creating tension in the neck muscles by lifting the head too high. It should feel as if it just floats up naturally, rather than being pulled up stiffly. Remember: muscles do not work efficiently when stretched.
- From the soles of the feet to the top of the head, eliminate rigidity and adopt an upright but flexing posture. Use a mirror to check your posture from the front and the side.
- As the head lifts, ensure that the knees are kept straight, loose and held in the middle (not pulled too far back or bent forward). This will help release the buttocks and pelvis and open up the core muscles of the spine and torso, allowing the joints and organs to breathe.

2. **Sink the shoulders and the elbows.**
Gradually relaxing the shoulders allows them to find their natural angle of repose, which visually is seen as falling or sloping away from the base of the neck. A body infused with tension draws in on itself, lifting and shortening the muscle fibres, recognized by raised or hunched-up shoulders. In this position the Qi becomes trapped and stagnant, floating high in the upper body and causing physical (especially in the heart and lungs) and emotional problems.

In order to settle the shoulders in the correct position the chest has to be "centered" (see Tai Chi Classic 3) and the elbows need to be placed to the side of the body, with the elbow-tips angled away from the body. This releases the armpits and centres the shoulder joints, allowing the Qi to flow unabated in and out of the arms and throughout the chest, upper back and shoulder girdle generally.

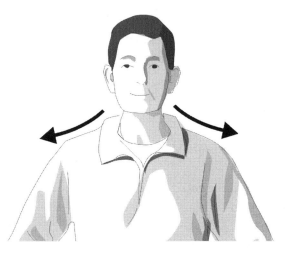

FIGURE 3: Natural Angle of Shoulder

NOTES

- Never force the shoulders or elbows down thinking it will develop instant "sinking". All that will be achieved is to tense the muscles and joints even more and restrict the breathing.
- The correct procedure is to first lift and centre the head gently at the Baihui crown point of the head. Then allow the elbows and shoulders to settle with the same sensitivity, lightness and gentleness of a feather falling to the earth.

3. **Hollow the chest and raise the upper back.**
   This is the much misunderstood Classic described earlier. Its title can be misleading; it obviously asks you to hollow the chest, and doing so raises the upper back. But the key is that the chest and the back should not remain fixed in this position; instead they should vacillate in a smooth and controlled manner between concave (Yang) and convex (Yin) posturing (see Figure 4).

   Between these two extremes, at the centre, lies the "Middle Path", the gravitational centre for the chest, upper body and spine. If the natural repose of the shoulders means they sit centrally in their sockets when at rest, then the natural repose of the chest means it should also sit centrally when at rest.

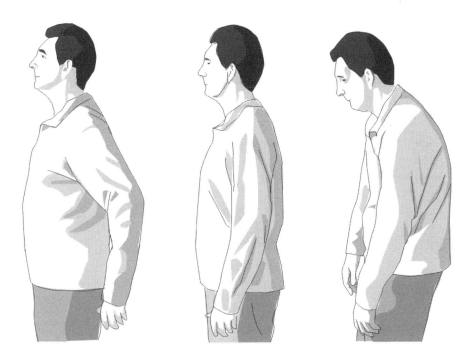

FIGURE 4: The Three Chest Positions

NOTES

- The general rule to sinking the Qi downwards to create a strong root through the feet is to release air from the lungs as you gradually lower the chest (Hollowing). To raise the Qi upwards, making the body feel light and agile, you must draw air into the lungs as you gradually lift the chest. To stand still and remain balanced, you must allow the chest to naturally centre itself. While in this posture, breathe gently through the nose and observe how this creates a natural swaying action that is centred in the chest (see Figure 4).
- Hollowing the chest is also called "Drawing the Bow", when applied with martial intent; and it is sometimes referred to as "Condensing the Qi" into the bones.
- Lifting the chest after hollowing it is called "Releasing the Arrows". This refers to the Qi arrows that were stored in the "Bow" of the spine flowing outwards through the arms and hands.

4. Loosen the waist and droop the buttocks.

To *loosen the waist* means in practical terms releasing the lower back muscles and hips through their full ROM (Range of Movement). In order to create this freedom of movement, time must be spent looking at the potential of what the Chinese call the "Qua". This is the line that runs from the hip joint along the crease where the thigh joins the torso at the lower abdomen and groin (see Figure 5) – known as the "Secret Fold". When the Qua is released (opening and closing of the fold), the Qi can freely circulate in and out of the legs, keeping the hips, knees and feet healthy.

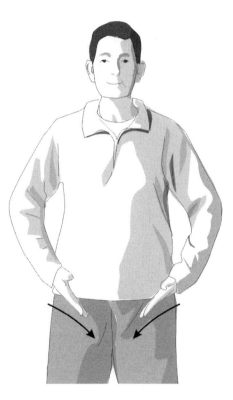

FIGURE 5: The Qua

To *droop the buttocks* means releasing the lumbar joints of the lower back. This is achieved by focusing on the Wei Lu cavity, situated on the coccyx at the tip of the spine, and allowing it to hang or "droop" down naturally. This has the effect, when done in conjunction with the Baihui, of opening up the joints of the spine (see Figure 6), encouraging its natural curvature.

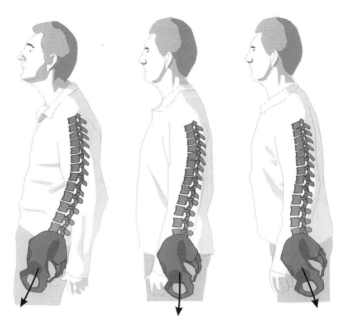

FIGURE 6: Pelvic Balance

NOTES

- The combined effects of loosening the waist and drooping the buttocks are designed to allow the pelvis to self-centre in the correct position, especially when the body comes to rest. To operate freely at the heart of all physical actions, the pelvis must have unrestricted turning (swivelling) and tilting (pivoting) ability.
- To regulate and normalize the pelvis, it is essential to keep the knees loose and relaxed and aligned correctly (they should be centred when standing straight).
- It is recommended to experiment with the three main axis points of mechanical motion in the body: knees, hips and centre of chest. They all influence each other in a positive and negative way: for example, the chest dictates the position of the pelvis and vice versa. The same is true of the knees and the pelvis.

"When turning, one must take care to keep the Wei Lu point and spine in alignment, in order to avoid losing Central Equilibrium."
— *CHEN MAN-CHING*

This is one of the many gems in this book that I recommend you take note of. An upright spine and naturally hung and centred pelvis help maintain stability when turning, and are especially valuable as we get older and find ourselves more prone to falls. *A further note:* make sure you turn with the head leading the waist (pelvis), both working together to retain your Central Equilibrium.

5. **All movements commence in the feet and materialize in the hands.**
   The fifth Classic is designed to delicately weave a Middle Path through all the joints and supporting tissues of the body. This is achieved by first uniting all the actions of the four previous maxims and then, in line with Newton's Law, by applying a downward force (gravity + natural body weight) through the soles of the feet, an equal upward counter-force will be produced. It is this upward resultant force, if harnessed and directed centrally through the joints, that will materialize visually (Jing) as a weaving and coiling "Body Wave", about which another linked Classic states:

"It commences in the feet and bursts forth in the fingers."

NOTES

- The ancient Chinese said that sensitivity is needed to direct the Wave through the body; it should be as light and delicate as the force necessary to draw a fine silken thread off the cocoon made by the silkworm. Too much force and the thread will snap, too little and it cannot be drawn. Therefore, the perfect force is the Middle Path frequency.
- As this force (Qi) rises up through the body it can be led by the eyes and focused mind (Yi) to "see" where you wish it to go (usually the distant horizon) and to visualize the same. This is what the ancient Chinese described as "Releasing Negative Qi". Dr John Tanner (orthopaedic and sports medicine), makes reference to the wave-like actions intrinsic to Tai Chi and Qigong motion when he recommends:

"Rhythmic action for chronic muscular tension."

The Qigong Classics

The source of these classics remains obscure; however, they have been documented in the book *Chinese Qigong Therapy* by Zhang Mingwu and Sun Xingyuan. As with their Tai Chi counterparts, they are interested in detailing correctness of posture, but with a slight twist: they describe in more detail how one part of the body structure influences another.

1. **Placing the feet shoulder-width apart, with weight evenly spread, takes undue pressure off the waist.**

   This posture maxim stresses the importance of positioning the feet on the earth in a way that transmits balanced structural support between the earth and the pelvis (see Figure 7). Even when the weight is spread evenly between both feet, whether the pelvis (waist) remains structurally balanced depends on your foot position.

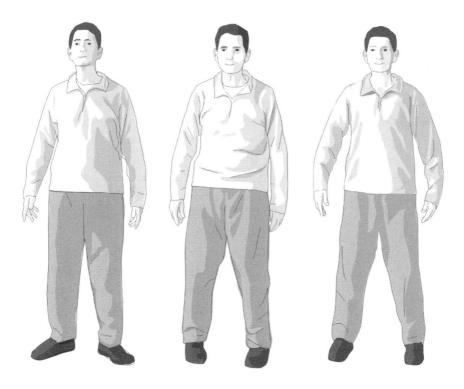

FIGURE 7: Feet to Body Alignment (Three Positions)

NOTES

- The image on the left is the most common fault. It distorts the gravity line to earth through the instep arches of both feet. This causes an inward "leaking" or collapsing of the foot arches, knees and hip joints. It also excessively opens the front of the body, tilting the pelvis backward and stiffening the back.
- The middle image has the opposite effect, causing an outward leaking to the outside edges of the feet, knees and hips. It also tilts the pelvis forward, excessively opens the back of the body and stiffens the front.
- In the desired and preferred image, on the right, the weight is not only even in both feet, but also spread evenly front to back between the heels and the toes to engage the "Bubbling Well" (Yongchuan) points. These are the gravitational centres of the feet, where the gravity line should naturally exit the body to earth (without any leakage on its journey down through the structural joints).
- The feet must point forward (especially the instep); this enables the structural load-bearing sections of the legs to align correctly all the way up to the pelvis and onward up through the spine.

2. **A relaxed knee joint helps improve the flow of Qi through the joint. It releases the hips, balances the pelvic girdle and loosens the whole waist.**
So many people live with tension trapped in their knees, without realizing the effect it is having on their posture and health. Tense knees radiate tension directly up and into the pelvic girdle, causing stiffness in the supporting tissues and throwing the pelvis out of alignment.

NOTES

- When held tense, the knees are restricted from operating through their full ROM. If the knees are fixed in a bent position, they make the upper body and spine slump; alternatively, if the knees are locked into a stiff upright position (pulled back against the joints – known as the ligament wall), the spine will do the same and become too stiff and upright.
- The knees should at all times be kept supple and moving through their full ROM. This should be achieved by exercising both when the knees

are loaded (standing, squatting, walking and running) and non-loaded (with the weight off the knees: sitting, lying down, or standing on one leg to flex the knee joint of the other leg).

- The knees are the centre of gravity of the legs and therefore influence all leg actions, including the legs' general health.
- The action of the knees increases the flow of power through the whole body, by accelerating the upward Yang force and downward Yin force.
- The knees also act as shock absorbers in the active body, which means they can de-accelerate the harmful forces that flow through the body.
- When at rest in an upright standing position, the knees should be held centrally, not bent forward or pulled backward against the ligament wall.

3. **When the hips are released, the lower limbs will move freely.**
   Ask anyone who has experienced any form of degeneration in the hip joint, "How did this affect your physical life?" They would all reply with one voice: "Dramatically!" This may be stating the obvious, but it does help highlight the importance of hip maintenance. Correct exercise and nutrition help to maintain the health of all the body's joints as well as is possible for as long as is possible; but the reality of a public uninformed on the fundamentals of self-healing and maintenance has developed into a major burden on the UK's National Health Service, where there is an ever-increasing demand for hip and knee replacements. We all can and should release the hips to enjoy the freedom of movement our legs are built to offer, and therefore lead a healthy, active life well into old age.

NOTES

- Misalignment of the structural frame, which includes the neck joints, can inadvertently create undue pressure on hip and knee joints. Therefore, start your structural corrections at the head and work down the spine to the pelvis to be kind to these joints.
- A major cause of undue wear and tear on the hips is the legs interacting incorrectly with the pelvis when bending and squatting (see Figure 10, page 56). For correct positioning of the pelvis when bending/squatting, see Figure 30, 1–4 Method, page 119.
- There are a number of simple hip exercises that take only a few minutes to perform, but make a major difference in the care and healthy

functioning of the hip joints. A visit to your local qualified Tai Chi and Qigong instructor will expose you to a range of these exercises.

- Walking using the full swing of the hips, known as "Natural Extended Stride Pattern" (see Chapter 7, Middle Path Walking) will help ward off stiffness and stagnation in the hips.

4. **To relax the waist, bend the knees and open the hips. When the waist is relaxed, the spine will stand upright but remain relaxed.**
This maxim deals with natural centring of the pelvis and how a centred pelvis can influence the spine. If the muscles in and around the pelvis are unnaturally tense, this tension gravitates both upward and downward. Upward tension restricts the diaphragm and chest cavity from naturally opening and closing. In addition, the spinal column becomes stiff and rigid due to the normally relaxed long muscles being held in tension.

This Classic is illustrated in Figure 8, where the desired posture on the left releases pelvic tension, but as you move to the right you can see the knee positions recreating the locked-up damaging stiffness, trapping the Qi high in the chest. However, when the waist is relaxed and therefore is able to "self-centre", the Qi is allowed to gravitate down to the Dan Tien and the earth as seen in Figure 6, page 33. A tense and locked pelvis (I call it "Frozen Girdle") will also gravitate a distortion down into the knees through the femur, thigh and hip flexor muscles, materializing as knee pain, often in the patella (kneecap).

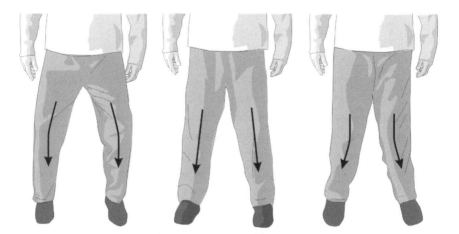

FIGURE 8: Three Knee Positions

Figure 8 shows how the knee position can be affected by pelvic posture. To create a strong root connection with earth, swing to the left. To weaken the stabilizing connection with the earth, swing to the right.

NOTES

- The pelvis must not be placed; it should with the help of the knees and chest be sensed and left to find its own level, like water.
- To release the waist and hips the knees should be bent only slightly, as if sitting on a horse, with the feet shoulder-width apart. The lower back and the spine generally should remain straight and not incline forwards (again see Figure 30, Upright Squat, page 119).
- When breathing out and lowering the shoulders to help relax the waist, consciously open the armpits a little to allow the torso and shoulder muscles (and Qi) to gravitate down naturally.

5. Chest tucking-in stretches the back muscles. Vertebrae tucking-in opens the ribs.
This health maxim states what the Tai Chi Classics do not: that to keep the spine, core muscles and organs of the torso (especially the heart and lungs) in good working order, the "Middle Mountain" (Shan Zhong cavity) must continually fluctuate between concave (chest tucking-in) and convex (vertebrae tucking-in). Together, this rhythmic action naturally regulates the heart and lungs, and creates more spaciousness in the thoracic (chest) cavity.

NOTES

- In order to lift and lower the Middle Mountain correctly through its full ROM, the pelvis must be activated to coordinate with and influence the chest movement. To lift the chest, the Wei Lu or Earth point, on the coccyx, the tailbone at the tip of the pelvis, must tilt backwards and outwards. To lower the chest the Wei Lu swings down and tucks under towards the front.
- The natural rise and fall of the chest cavity regulates the breathing: Vertebrae tucking-in = inhalation; Chest tucking-in = exhalation.
- When the body is at rest, for example sitting down or standing still, the chest should be maintained in an upright but central position

(neither convex nor concave). In this position, when you inhale and exhale the torso will rise and fall. This is natural and should not be constricted in any way.

- As respiration is the most essential body function for life, it is worth noting the four fundamental body parts for healthy breathing: abdominal cavity, diaphragm, chest cavity and airways.

6. **Back-stretching means to let the vertebrae stand upright in the Middle.**
This "back-stretching" is a cryptic way of describing how to achieve perfect upright posture with the spine at its core (see Figure 4, page 31). This is also known in the Tai Chi world as "Wu Chi", which means "No Extremity" or Middle Path; not too straight and not too bent, but halfway between the two: upright and straight but with relaxed natural curves.

NOTES

- When the body is at rest, as described in Note 3 to the previous Classic, the pelvis, like the chest, should be maintained in a central position (not tucked under, or tilted out). The coordination of movement between pelvis and chest remains, but is more subtle and less visibly obvious.
- The intimate interaction between the pelvis and the chest cavity, in a torso that is structurally well aligned, creates perfect conditions for the diaphragm to operate to its maximum efficiency.
- Wu Chi describes the overall Energy Body (Jinglo) condition of a physically centred and upright body bathed in stillness (see Chapter 6).

7. **The natural drooping of the shoulders relaxes the neck. To droop the shoulders it is necessary to hollow the armpits. When the shoulders are naturally drooping and the armpits are maintained, the Qi and the blood in the upper limbs will flow more easily.**
It is interesting to note how in this maxim the importance of hollowing the armpits is stressed. The reason for hollowing the armpits is to open the shoulder structure (the joints and supporting soft tissues), which encourages the shoulder generally to naturally drop.

NOTES

- When the armpits are maintained open but not fixed, the chest cavity can expand and contract due to the shoulders being open and the arms being kept away from touching the body.
- When a person is carrying tension, it manifests in the shoulders by contracting the trapezius and pectoral muscles, which pulls the shoulders both upward and inward, causing compression on the neck. Therefore, when the same person is relaxed, the shoulders are meant to fall away from the spine (see Figure 3, page 30), thus releasing the pressure on the neck.
- It is important to note, when directing the shoulders to where they should naturally reside, that this can only be fully achieved by locating the elbows correctly (naturally open and in the middle). The elbows are the root of the shoulders.

8. **Keep the head as if it were suspended. When suspended, the head must be kept in the Middle. An upright head is the key to settling the whole body in an upright position. A centred head nourishes the brain and invigorates the spirit.**
It is interesting how the Qigong Classics place this last in the list, when it is clearly the most important of them all. The head is the command centre of the body; it directs all operations including positioning of the structural frame. It connects to the top of the spine and therefore when it lifts, the spine lifts. Conversely, when it sags, the spine sags.

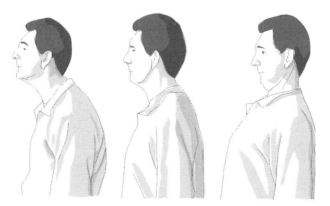

FIGURE 9: The Three Head Positions

NOTES

- The head should not be locked into one position when suspended; just like the chest and pelvis, it is meant to rise and fall with the respiratory action.
- When the head is linked mechanically with the chest and pelvis the following resultant actions take place: pelvis to chest = opening of the diaphragm. Chest to head = opening of the chest cavity and airways. Pelvis to chest to head = opening of the spine and organs.
- The upright centred head nourishes the brain, for two main reasons: with the head placed in the Middle the blood vessels are performing like hosepipes free from kinks; and, with an efficiently working respiratory system, the oxygenated blood is delivered to the organ that demands the most oxygen, namely the brain. The increased level of oxygen intake and more efficient carbon expulsion raise the energy levels, which invigorates the spirit.
- The position you hold your head in, bearing in mind its weight (typically eight to twelve pounds), is of great importance to the healthy functioning of everything that lies beneath.

Questions and Answers

Isn't the Classics just common sense?

Of course it is; it is quite simply nature's common sense for the human body. Problems occur because the majority of people don't adhere to her (nature's) laws, which are:

1. Align the body correctly with gravity.
2. Sustain good posture in stillness and in motion.
3. Listen to your inner regulator voice, that tells you when to: drink, eat, urinate, defecate, sleep, play, work and rest.

The Classics are designed to help us achieve numbers 1 and 2 above and by doing so create number 3.

I am finding there are too many things to do all at once, which only leaves me frustrated.

This is because you may be trying too hard to create instant perfect posture. You will note that the Classics have been written in the form of a descending sequence that starts at the head and progressively works its way down through the body, correcting posture as it goes. I suggest you start with this and do it one step at a time, for example:

1. Spend a week just gently lifting the crown of the head to realign the neck, observing how this lifts the spine and helps centre the chest and shoulders.
2. After this, start working on the shoulders and retain what should now be a better-aligned head position.
3. Now lift and roll the shoulders forwards and backwards in harmony with lifting and lowering the centre of the chest, to release the whole upper body.
4. Continue with this until you have progressed through all the directions of the five Tai Chi Classics.
5. The next step is to go back over the whole body, but this time in accord with the Qigong Classics, from the feet upwards.

Why does my body feel stiff when I am in the positions described?
It sounds as though you are holding the shapes instead of moving and living with them. The shapes described represent a body at rest (sitting or standing), but it is important to note that you should extend your body forward of the centre when stretching upwards and backward of the centre when bending. By doing this, you are exercising your body correctly (see Chapter 6) and not holding it stiffly at the centre, where it should only be when you come to rest (upright and still).

I am in my late sixties and have not been posture-aware. I am quite bent over and I have been told I have early-stage osteoporosis. How can I straighten my spine without doing myself damage?
Many people who attend my classes are living with varying degrees of osteoporosis and because of the nature of the disease, I keep a particularly close eye on how they are performing the therapies. They all have a weakened structure and tend to stoop, which impacts even more on the degeneration of the spine. I therefore teach them to take the focus off their bones and concentrate on the soft tissues that support the structural frame. If you try to straighten the spine using the bones, you run the risk of further bone damage; however, if you relax, realign and move through the supporting soft tissues instead, you will improve your posture safely. The circulation around the joints will improve and the damaging gravitational force that accompanies drooped posture will be directed away from the joints.

This makes a dramatic difference to the quality of life of osteoporosis sufferers; they generally find that they can now move with a freedom and confidence that they had not enjoyed since before the onset of the disease.

EXPERIENCE IN PRACTICE

1. Relax the whole body by gentle shaking, flexing and extending.

2. "Feel" the connection your feet have with the spine by lowering your body to "Earth" (see Figure 12 , page 73) through the knees. Then push gently upwards from the ground to lift your torso and spine up. Fuel the whole cyclic process with gentle nose-breathing (Inhale – up. Exhale – down).

3. Link the chest to this up and down total-body motion by becoming aware of the chest naturally rising as part of this rising wave and sensing how it naturally falls like an autumn leaf on the downward cycle.

3

Middle Path Posture for Healthy Balance

"Though heaven frown and earth darken, neither sun nor storm,
lightning nor rain can cause me to lose my way.
Though my journey through life be full of danger and hardship,
I stay safely on the 'Middle Path'."
— *KO HUNG*

The vital linkage between posture and health is finally dawning on those involved in Western medicine; but it is still not being talked about enough at grassroots level. The plain facts are that posture has a major influence on the health of an individual; in this chapter we will examine the negative aspects of postural defects and discover what damage they cause.

"Posture degeneration starts in the feet. Therefore look to the feet to rectify the problem."
— *ANCIENT CHINESE MAXIM*

In Traditional Chinese Medicine (TCM), postures are categorized as being "Yin", "Yang" or "Middle Path", with all three having a profound effect on the well-being of the individual. Generally, Yin postures are defined as when the front (Yin) of the body tends to collapse or slump downwards, causing the back (Yang) of the body to bend forward. In contrast, a Yang posture is when the front of the body is unnaturally extended upwards and outwards, causing the back (spine) to overextend inwards, creating the classic "lean back" posture. The definition of a Middle Path posture is when Yin and Yang are operating in perfect harmony within the structural frame. Before we embark on the posture analysis contained in this chapter it is worth noting the following observation:

"For every one inch that the head is out of alignment, the muscles and joints of the spine and pelvis are subjected to 25 pounds of excess stress."
— *DR ROBERT SIMMONS*, **Chiropractic and Kinesiology Centre, Charlotte, USA**

Excessive Yin Posture

This posture type (see Figure 10, page 56) is usually associated with conditions such as ankylosing spondylitis, Parkinson's disease and osteoporosis. But more often than not, it appears as a result of slouching, caused by a lack of postural awareness. The negative physical effects on the body are:

- Damaging lordosis of the lower neck vertebra, caused by the head and neck extending forward.
- Uneven and excessive wear and tear on the vertebral discs.
- Compression of the torso muscles at the front and overextension of the muscles at the back.
- Restricted range of movement of the shoulders, caused by them being shunted too far forward.
- Compression and restriction of the diaphragm and chest cavity.
- Compression and restriction of the organs.
- Misalignment of the pelvis (tucked too far under).
- Knees unnaturally bent, even when the body is standing still.
- Arms tending to fall in to touch the sides of the body, closing the armpits and restricting chest cavity expansion.
- Misplacement of hip joints, limiting their range of movement.
- The body's weight is gravitated to the heels, limiting the natural heel-to-toe rolling walking action of the underside of the feet, creating heel walking (see "Yin Heel Walkers", Chapter 7).
- All the joints of the body become stiffer, creating the ideal conditions for arthritis.
- Oxygen supply to the cells drops and carbon retention increases.
- Skin texture sags and weakens and the complexion becomes sallow, due to the likely presence of hypotension (low blood pressure).
- The gravitational core drops down and back and disturbs the general equilibrium of the body.
- The voice noticeably loses its power and projection.
- Emotionally, this posture suppresses the Living Spirit.

This is obviously a most undesirable posture. Generally it develops over many years and is allowed to develop because people lack postural awareness and are simply unaware of the damage they are doing to themselves.

NOTES OF CAUTION

- Before commencing with the posture corrections (for both this and Excessive Yang posture), it is recommended you discuss your intentions with your doctor to ensure that there are no medical reasons why you should not do so.
- It is advised you only attempt the corrections under the guidance of a qualified Tai Chi or Qigong instructor, especially if you have any underlying health conditions.
- When adjusting the spine and joints generally to improve posture, all movements must be practised slowly, gently and gradually. Do not force the joints into positions they are unable to achieve or hold.

Excessive Yin Body Correction

To realign your posture, there are five key structural changes: the head crown point (Baihui), the chest centre point (Shan Zhong), the abdomen centre (Qi Hai), the knees generally and the feet (Yongchuan).

1. **The Head Crown Point:** This according to the ancient Chinese is the Baihui, "The One Hundred Convergences" point, meaning that at this point on the head the body's meridians (lines of power, like ley lines) converge with the point of entry for gravity. When the Crown Point remains centred, everything below becomes centred; the structural physical body and the Energy Body (Jinglo) become aligned.

    To correct a misaligned head, lift the Crown Point up at the same time as gently pulling the chin in and you will notice the neck vertebrae straightening up, allowing the eyes to level out on the distant horizon.

2. **The Chest Centre Point:** This is known as the Middle Mountain and influences the spine just as does the tallest mountain in a mountain range. To correct a slumping spine, the Middle Mountain must be lifted upward at all times, but while simultaneously remembering that upward means "to the middle", not excessively lifted.

3. **Abdomen Centre:** This is the centre of gravity for the whole body and therefore it stands to reason that this centre holds influence over all body-motion. When the abdomen centre is level and parallel to the earth, it dictates that the other centres of motion also become level and even. Therefore, pointing the navel directly forward (not angled down or up) helps to achieve this. To reposition and release the Yin-fixed, excessively tilted-under pelvis, the chest centre (Shan Zhong) should when standing be moved up and down in conjunction with a coccyx that swings back and forth. As a result of this the pelvic girdle will begin to move freely and the navel will naturally level out to reflect a balanced pelvis.

4. **The Knees:** As these are the centre of gravity for the legs their location has a direct impact on the hips, which are in turn responsible for positioning the pelvis. In this posture, the knees are usually left in a bent position, even when the individual thinks they are standing upright (see "Beware the False Brain" below). This, over time, results in reducing the ROM of the knees, restricting physical motion and creating the perfect conditions for arthritis. The knees project the energy rising from the feet upwards into the pelvis and spine. To lift the centre line of the torso up from its slouching position, the knees should be not only straightened to align the leg vertically, but should also be encouraged to flex backwards (gently) against the ligament wall. The effect of this is to tilt the pelvis outward, to thrust the chest and head upwards, stretching and opening the core tissues.

5. **The Feet:** Most people with an Excessive Yin posture will have their gravitational centre moved back along the foot into the heels, caused by the spine bowing out excessively towards the back. In order to provide the force necessary to lift the spine back into place, we must look to the feet. In the centre of foot sole, at the base of the ball of the foot lies the important energy cavity known as the Yongchuan, which means "Bubbling Well". This is the gravity centre of the foot and where the gravity line of the whole body communicates with the earth. To deliver the upward rising power that moves the key centres mentioned above into their correct structural positions, the feet must be spread evenly on the earth.

An important point to note at this juncture is that the rising connective and corrective power must be derived from feet that are pointing perfectly forward. This unifies the resultant upward force and allows it to flow through correctly aligned bones, joints, muscles, ligaments and tendons. The moving Jing (energy) must be centred and flow gently, otherwise joint and tissue damage may result. Therefore, to achieve the above, the initial downward-focused push action through the feet must be sensed to enter the earth through the Yongchuan.

In the Western world when we desire to push something with great force away from the body, we engage the heels with the earth and tense the body's muscles. This delivers the required power to the hands – classed as "External" power. True or "Internal" power comes only from the Yongchuans, which move the gravity line out of the spine and forward into the torso centre, engaging the soft tissues, to a position the ancient Chinese call the "Tai Zhong Mai" (Central Channel, see Figure 11, page 61).

Excessive Yang Posture

Yang is linked to heaven and the element of fire, meaning the Qi, posture and emotions (spirit) gravitate upwards to excess, if not controlled by the balancing force of Yin. A typical Excessive Yang posture would be a body that has its central core unnaturally raised upward and forward, a position that causes general stagnation, especially in the upper body. As with the Excessive Yin posture, it is often caused by a lack of postural awareness. Here are some of the negative effects on the mind, body and spirit of this posture:

- With the gravity core shunted forward, the head tends to pull back in excess to compensate, causing a stiff erect neck.
- The extended Middle Mountain spine-centre causes the spine and organs to be misplaced (shunted forward).
- The shoulders are thrown back off centre, which compresses the muscles between the shoulder blades and the spine, and plants the seeds of frozen shoulder.
- It is common for the whole shoulder girdle to elevate upward, which impacts directly on the lower neck vertebrae.
- With the lungs being pushed forward against the ribs and the diaphragm stressed, high chest breathing ensues. This is caused by the lungs not being able to expand and contract equally in the centre of the chest cavity, seriously interfering with the respiration of oxygen and carbon.
- The loading on the vertebral discs becomes uneven, tending to compress the outward facing edge of the joints on mid and lower spine

and inward facing on the neck. This unequal loading creates perfect conditions for the discs to suffer prolapses.

- The pelvis is held in a permanent state of forward tilt, which overextends the abdominal muscles and compresses the lower back muscles and creates excessive lordosis of the lumbar spine.
- The hips are thrown back and outwards from where they should naturally reside, in the centre of the housing sockets.
- The knees are constantly held against the rear ligament wall, creating undue wear and tear on the cartilage and perfect conditions for osteoarthritis.
- The gravity line is thrown into the ball of the foot and toes, which impacts on the natural heel-to-toe rolling action of the foot and produces tiptoe walking instead. This makes the gait unsteady and stiffens the legs, so they cannot flex as efficiently and naturally as they should.
- All the body's joints are liable to grow stiff, due to excessively tensed muscles. Perfect conditions for raised blood pressure (hypertension).
- The skin is flushed and red due to this self-induced hypertension.
- The voice is chesty, loud and gravelly.
- Emotionally, Yang people tend to be short-tempered and poor listeners.
- The combination of organ displacement and fiery temperament damages the natural balance of the digestive system.

Excessive Yang Body Correction

Numerous health-impairing conditions can arise from perpetuating this posture. The longer these structural deformities remain the more damage they cause; if this postural condition sounds like you, you can follow the guidance notes below:

1. Place both hands over the Qi Hai point (25mm below the navel), pull the abdominal wall back from within on an exhalation and coordinate a pulling inward action with the hands. This will straighten the abdominal wall, centre the pelvis and create equilibrium throughout all the lower torso muscles.

2. The chest centre (Middle Mountain) will now naturally lower itself and should level off facing the horizon. This centres the chest cavity, enabling it to expand and contract equally with each respiration cycle.

3. The knees will drop forward and relocate to the centre of the joints, allowing the pelvis to hinge upward to its required level position.

4. The head will naturally release itself to raise up slightly to its home centre. This releases the vice-like grip of the rear neck muscles, leaving a neck with natural curvature.

5. The shoulders, which should by nature be self-levelling, will drop down and fall forward to the centre of their housing sockets. This opens the armpits, enabling free-flowing Qi to journey in and out of the limbs.

6. The pelvis, like the shoulders, is meant to be self-adjusting/levelling; providing it regains its full range of movement (ROM), it will automatically keep its centred posture in the future.

"With height increased, cut back its peak to
make the mountain stable."
— *I CHING*

This ancient gem from the *I Ching* states in eloquent abbreviation how to find the perfect posture. "Rectify the Excessive Yin and Yang and return the body to the middle." And here is the *I Ching's* secret to finding the physical Middle Path:

Stand and stretch up through the core as you breathe in, to create an 'Excessive Yang' sinew-stretching posture (with height increased). Now lower the body a little as you breathe out (cut back its peak) and feel the whole body 'settle' in a centred upright posture (to make the mountain stable).

Posture and Health Guidance

"Let no part of your movements indicate imperfection,
neither over-expanded or caving in."
— *CHANG SAN FENG*

Prevention of Falls

At the time of writing this book, it was reported that in the UK alone an average of 11,000 elderly people are admitted to hospital each year directly as a result of falling (it is over two million in the USA). The cost of treatment and aftercare probably runs into tens of millions of pounds and the frustrating thing is that a high proportion of these falls could probably be avoided if everybody over fifty followed a programme of Tai Chi and Qigong exercises. Here are some more painful statistics to consider:

Every year, one in three people over sixty-five have a serious fall. Falls can cause loss of confidence, which may affect older people's independence and cause social isolation. Falls are the biggest cause of accidental death in the UK. Every five hours an older person dies after a fall at home. *(Source – Help the Aged)*

So what can be done? The first thing to do is lobby your doctor to provide access to a qualified registered Tai Chi and Qigong instructor, a person who could offer the benefits reported in the many scientific studies undertaken by reputable medically trained experts in the field (see Chapter 9). Here are the key benefits that Tai Chi and Qigong offer to help prevent falls:

1. **Structural Reprogramming:** The human body relies for good health and performance on being structurally aligned with gravity, which is why this is intrinsic to the training, in the form of posture corrections to achieve the shapes described and shown in the Tai Chi and Qigong Classics (see Chapter 2).

2. **Proprioception:** is the neuromuscular feedback system of balance awareness throughout the body that has a tendency to degenerate in later life, if not nurtured and maintained. Tai Chi and Qigong mechanics stimulate this electrical bio-sensory system and keep it activated well into old age, thus reducing the potential for falls.

3. **The Three Stabilizers:** By placing our awareness on the Baihui crown point on the *head*, freeing up the *waist and hips* and sensing the Yong-chuan gravitational centres of the *feet*, the body can and does develop its Central Equilibrium. This ensures that the body moves with grace and balance, free from the uneven loading of joints and muscles that restricts balance, circulation and coordination.

4. **To Move Through the Tendons:** Another important point to consider is the unique way Tai Chi and Qigong practitioners move with awareness on the tendons and other soft tissues of the body. The bones offer us a core structure for good posture, but it is our soft tissues that motorize it for healthy body-mechanics.

Those who move their bodies with their attention (albeit subconscious)
on the bones, move with awkwardness, stiffness and impaired balance.
Those who move through the tendons retain the balance and suppleness
of a child. Don't carry your body, Let your body carry you.
— *P T N*

It is easy to copy

Beware falling into the trap of just becoming a carbon copy; it is possible to super-ficially adopt a good posture but retain postural stiffness. The way to adopt healthy posture is to feel its shape as an internal expression. Sense its presence, in stillness and in motion, by becoming aware of your Jinglo (energy body). Through this method you will develop the important subconscious muscle memory.

Beware the false brain

People who have been away from their home centre for a considerable time, with excessive Yin or Yang posture, can develop a "false brain". This in practical terms means that the neurosensory feedback system of the body, the proprio-ceptors, become confused. With the body being out of alignment for so long, the brain begins to believe the incorrect is correct. This is apparent whenever I centre a person who for many years has lived with excessive Yin or Yang posture. The comment is usually, "I feel like I am leaning too far back" (for a Yin posture person), or "I feel I am leaning to far forwards" (for a Yang posture person). They then go on to talk of feeling so unsteady they are nervous they may topple over, and when they are returned back to their incorrect posture they comment "Ahh… that feels better."

"Do not confuse the true with the false. Recognize the difference
between the human mind and the mind of Dao. Do not mistake the
false body for the true body."
— *T'AI SHANG LAO-CHUN (LAO-TSU)*

"YOUR BODY" Principle

To help people gain an understanding of the benefits of becoming posture-conscious, I have devised the "Your Body" Principle. This offers a succinct life guide on the essentials to enjoy a healthy Middle Path life.

"Y"

When people are told they are "old" or "elderly", or when the doctor tells them the reason why they are becoming stiff is "because of your age", they believe it. By believing, they are in fact supporting the decline in the physical dexterity of their own bodies: "They say I'm old, therefore I must be." To counter this self-defeating belief, it is essential to disengage from conforming normality and instead embrace your inner child spirit. This reintroduces the spirit of vitality to cells in the body and brain that thought they had gone into retirement. "Y", therefore, represents a "Youthful Mind and Outlook".

"O"

In order for a misaligned posture to be corrected by self-directed conscious action, it must first be physically conditioned to be able to achieve what you are asking of it. The physical structural body is made up in a subtle balance of hard (skeletal frame) and soft (muscles, tendons, ligaments) tissues. Unless homeostasis exists between the hard and the soft, it is impossible to tune in to the invisible force of nature. A force that naturally self-levels and self-adjusts, to create structural balance. A tense body manifests through its soft tissues; tension originates in a stressed mind and therefore it is here that the road to a relaxed, self-adjusting body must start. "O", therefore, represents "Openness" between "Mind and Body".

"U"

When a hosepipe develops a kink and the flow of water becomes impaired, the only way to rectify the blockage is to straighten and stretch out the hose. In the human body exactly the same principle applies: for example, when you lie on your arm overnight and wake with pins and needles. The human form, due to evolution, demands to be held in an upright position while sitting, standing and walking and to deny the body this is to introduce blockages. Additionally, when any structure, including a body, is vertically upright it becomes structurally sound and able to move safely, reducing the potential for falling. "U", therefore, represents the "Upright" frame that is essential for good health and efficient body mechanics.

"R"

Although the body is now structurally centred, upright and relaxed, the picture is still not complete. There must be an additional dimension in order to achieve posture perfection: this is tension-free, structurally sound, comprehensive joint movement. Even if the hard frame is gravitationally aligned, if full joint stimulation is ignored the Qi will remain sluggish and locked in the muscles, tendons, ligaments and the joints. "R", therefore, represents the "Range" of joint movement that must be regularly explored.

"B"

When everything that gives the body shape is centred and settled in the optimum position for the mechanics of support and healthy motion to occur, other essential functions, such as circulation and respiration, are given a boost. The body is now free from internal conflict, giving the Dao unmitigated access to operate. This means, in Daoist medical terms, that the body can not only breathe with natural depth into the lungs, but also achieve the desired state of being known as "Grand Circulation" (whole body breathing). "B", therefore, represents "Breathing" to the maximum potential.

"O"

Regulated breathing is just one of the many vital body functions needed to sustain good health. All the organs of the body have their role, their function in the deeply sophisticated body mechanism. The lungs, diaphragm and chest cavity are only able to perform correctly if they are located and motorized where (and in the way) the Dao wants them to be. That obviously makes sense, but what is often overlooked is that exactly the same principles apply to all of the body's other organs. The bladder, sexual reproduction organs, small intestine, large intestine, kidneys, liver, gallbladder, spleen, pancreas, stomach, heart and lungs have to be maintained in their home locations in order for them to mutually communicate and individually function. "O", therefore, represents the "Organs" being retained in their place, whether the body is in motion or at rest.

"D"

A body that is upright, open, breathing and in tune with gravity releases its inbuilt self-levelling potential. A body that is directed by the Dao and free from stress and tension becomes self-regulating in respect of physical structure, internal circuitry and emotions. "D", therefore, represents the free and equal "Distribution" of weight across the whole structure that allows it to find its Central Equilibrium.

"Y"

According to the ancient Chinese, a body that is operating outside of the Middle Path is a body that has left home. By returning to the Dao both physically and emotionally, you have once again become a real person and only real people reside at home. "Y", therefore, represents "Yourself", for this is what you find when you return home to the Dao.

Sitting on the Pelvis

This is the best way to describe the postural condition of many people who, through lack of posture awareness, develop a collapsed slumped posture that sits directly down onto a misaligned pelvic girdle. Figure 10 offers a visual of this:

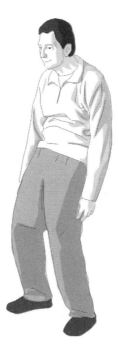

FIGURE 10: Sitting on the Pelvis - Not to Copy

This posture can have a devastating effect on the core muscles: the pelvic floor, multifidi spinae erectors, transverse abdominis, internal and external oblique. These collectively are the major muscles involved in keeping your torso straight and assisting in its correct bending. This is the worst of all negative postures the body can fall into, because of the damage it does to the organs, breathing, circulation, joints, physicality and emotions. For tips on how to address this see "Excessive Yin Posture", in Chapter 3.

Posture and Guardian Qi

The Guardian Qi is in a tangible sense, what we in the Western world call the immune system, that guards us against invading bacteria and viruses. Qi is nurtured and stored throughout autumn and winter, then transforms to Guardian Qi to help ward off what TCM considers the "windborne" diseases of spring. It relies on and is directly linked to good and natural posture, in stillness and motion.

Here are some more interesting facts on Guardian Qi:

Guardian Qi's Three Influential Meridians

The Small Heavenly Cycle is made up of the "Du Mai" or governor meridian, which is Yang in nature (see Figure 11, page 61) and the "Ren Mai", or conception meridian, which is Yin in nature. Together they form a harmonious circuit of Qi. Only when they are full of healthy Qi does the "Tai Zhong Mai" or central meridian assume its rightful place in the generation of Guardian Qi. While the three meridians all work to generate the Guardian Qi, it is the Du Mai, in the spine, that is richest in it. From here it is transported to the surface of the skin and beyond to form an aura-like glowing force field. Harmonizing the governor and conception meridians nourishes the brain and raises the Shen. The Shen when raised leads the Guardian Qi to the skin, which strengthens its shielding effect around the body. The conception meridian controls the distribution and dispersion of excess Guardian Qi across the abdomen and thorax, via the smaller subsidiary meridians. All of this intrinsically depends on good posture and "Huxi" (whole body breathing), in stillness and in motion.

Guardian Qi and Breathing

Supported by the respiratory function, the Guardian Qi is responsible for sweating and for opening and closing the skin's pores. According to Chinese Traditional Medicine Guardian Qi is Yang Qi and therefore represents the fire of the Five Elements. It is also involved in the regulation and control of body temperature. Through the development of Grand Circulation, where the whole body is opened and serviced by healthy Qi, the Guardian Qi is transported to the surface and forms a protective shield.

Guardian Qi will manifest only as a result of leading a sensible Middle Path lifestyle:

- Eating and drinking healthily.
- Avoiding addictive substances.
- Avoiding excessive sexual activity.
- Getting enough sleep and rest.
- Exercising regularly in a balanced and natural way.
- Awakening your inner consciousness.

Middle Path Posture "Settling"

This is another way in which the Chinese system emphasizes relaxing, but it is specifically used in the context of adopting the natural "Dao Posture". Anyone can strike a pose, but do they settle in that pose? The correct way to experience the Dao's self-healing "Formless Posture", in stillness and in motion, is to first stretch and enlarge the chosen shape to the individual's limit (on an in-breath), then settle (lower) the muscles, joints and structural frame (on an out-breath) so that you fall into the centre, where you will find the Middle Path.

The best method of experiencing this natural phenomenon is by using the "sideways coiling" method, which is accomplished by turning the head and waist left or right, with the feet fixed, shoulder-width apart, pointing forwards. Hold the twist to the side, then release the muscles. You will notice the body "uncoiling" naturally to return to facing front – this is settling. Middle Path Posture is not just physical; it flows into the realms of life and spirit:

Through kindness, compassion and caring
You find the Middle Path of Earth.

Through learning, patience and time
You find the Middle Path of knowledge.

Through life's experiences and virtue
You find the Middle Path of wisdom.

Through your inner cultivation and stillness
You find the Middle Path of Heaven.

Now Heaven and Earth coexist within you
And you walk the "Path" of the enlightened.

— P T N

As you can see, the Middle Path weaves its way through our lives, but it all starts with correctness of posture, which centres and strengthens the Qi at our core. Below is another Daoist representation of this principle:

The Three Ascending Paths of Immortality

YIN = Lesser Path = Earth = Body.

YIN/YANG = Middle Path = Human = Body/Mind/Spirit.

YANG = Greater Path = Celestial = Spirit.

Although there are three paths, there is only one Way. The one Way is the Dao. There are those who walk the Earth Path and look no further than the Body. The Middle Path walkers, however, are in possession of the essential Three needed to enter the realms of the Daoist goal, the Great Celestial Path. Lao-tsu comments on the Middle Path of the Dao when he states:

"It is the only way to conduct one's life."

Angle of Repose

This term is commonly used in structural engineering, but is also relevant here in regards to postural naturalness and correctness. In structural engineering, the angle of repose relates to the angle naturally formed by the outer sloping surface of, for example, sand, soil, gravel or wet concrete when tipped in a freestanding heap.

When the human body comes to rest, it too has natural angles of repose, which should be actively encouraged by doing Daoism's "Nothing". These special angles appear at various locations throughout the body: the head, along the shoulder-line, front and back of the chest, shoulder to elbow, elbow to wrist, pelvic girdle front and side elevations, hip to knee and knee to ankle.

Middle Path Core Posture

The first thing is to explain the Western understanding of the phrase "Core Posture"; the ancient Chinese understanding has some of the same features but is arguably deeper and more profound.

Western

In the West, the term "core posture" is typically used by professionals including physiotherapists, chiropractors, osteopaths and Pilates instructors. It is made up of the following key muscles that, together, unite to maintain our structural integrity:

1. **Pelvic Floor or Diaphragm.** This comprises the inner pelvic muscles that make up the functioning walls and floor of the bowl-shaped pelvic diaphragm. Below this is the perineum membrane, which supports the pelvic muscles from below.

2. **Transverse Abdominis.** This is the deepest layer of the three types of abdominal muscles (internal, external and transverse), and acts like a corset to the whole abdominal region including the pelvis.

3. **Multifidi.** These are the smallest and deepest layer of the back muscles that link each vertebra of the spine to the next. They form the rear portion of the structural core and support the length of the spine.

Chinese

This includes the above, but in addition encompasses two uniquely Chinese physical and spiritual concepts:

1. **Core Coordination.** This is the unification of the feet, knees, hips, pelvis, spine and head in an upward rising wave-like action that the ancients described as:

   "The unification of the 'Three Powers' (San Cai): Heaven, Earth and a gravitationally aligned and attuned human body."

The special coordination this produces unlocks our physical (muscular) and physiological (organ function and circulation) potential, driving them to their maximum efficiency. When the rising wave reaches the spine it "stacks" the joints, one by one on top of each other, until it reaches the top of the neck to create what is called "Full Extension". This benefits the cerebral spinal cord and stimulates surrounding cerebral fluid circulation and essential spine flexibility. The same can be said of when the body is at rest, where the soft rhythmic breathing function of lungs and diaphragm naturally rocks the torso back and forth, creating a mild extension and flexion of the spine. In a body that lacks core coordination, this important mutually supportive action between the core muscles and the lungs/diaphragm is impeded.

2. **Central Channel (Zhong Mai).** This is the home of the Shen and the actual gravitational core of the body (see Figure 11). It sits in the core of the torso in front of the spine and is said to manifest only when the physical body (spine and all core structural muscles) is perfectly aligned with the Dao (gravity) and core coordination is added. Its faint strands still remain in people who have developed posture problems, and the degree to which it is retrievable depends on the core condition and commitment of the individual. Its purest state is seen in very young children (up to about five years old) and when it returns in adults, you will have achieved what the Classics describe as "The softness and pliability of a child." If this channel is kept strong, all aspects of human physical, mental and spiritual health become equally strong.

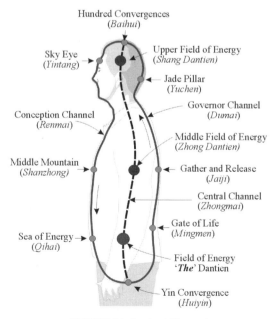

FIGURE 11: Central Channel

61

Middle Path Posture Summary

To summarize all the above:

- Left – Right, Forward – Backward, Up – Down, In – Out… so many directions and positions, but only one centre.
- The body naturally regulates itself, but only when it is centred.
- Balanced motion relies on the body operating through the centre.
- The body knows where everything in it should be; the centre encourages this.

A Middle Path "At Rest" centred posture would therefore be summarized as:

Head upright, crown point vertical,
eyes on distant horizon (By You).

Middle Mountain point of chest elevates
and points horizontally forward (By Dao).

Shoulders fall away from the neck
at the angle of repose (By Dao).

Shoulders, viewed from the side,
sit central on the upper torso (By Dao).

Knees straight, centred, consistently relaxed
and kneecaps pointing forward (By You).

Tailbone hanging down, pelvis level when still and free-swinging
and horizontally swivelling when in motion (By Dao).

~~⌐

Feet pointing perfectly straight, with weight spread
evenly across the soles (By Dao and By You).

KEY

By You = you create it and consistently ensure these conditions remain.

By Dao = nature sees to it, providing you have created the other conditions.

The motionless gravitationally centred body now has a home centre, where the
body, mind and spirit return to in stillness. This is the Middle Path.

> *"Excessive suppleness weakens, excessive tightness stiffens, Middle Path
> strengthens."*
> — *DAOIST AND BUDDHIST CONCEPT*

When in motion, the Middle Path gives the body a central reference point that
controls and regulates all intimate physical actions. This means the elimination of excesses: excessive extension = over-functioning; excessive contraction
= under-functioning. By the elimination of these excess forces we can achieve
Central Equilibrium (Zhong Pingheng), which manifests as:

> *Expansion and Contraction – Equalized.*
> *Raising and Lowering – Equalized.*
> *Opening and Closing – Equalized.*
> *Work to Life Balance – Equalized.*
> *Destructive Emotions – Equalized.*
> *Rampant and Passive Spirit – Equalized.*

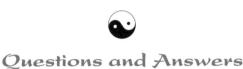

Questions and Answers

I have a classic Yin posture according to your guidance notes. Why doesn't it straighten up when I do as you instruct?

It depends on your age and how long you have been living with this posture. A young person (up to the age of about thirty) will find it much easier to reprogramme their core muscles. They will generally only take about six months to notice a major change to their posture, because younger muscle fibres are more pliable and adaptable to change. Once over about thirty, however, it takes progressively longer and longer for posture-damaged joint and muscle injuries to recover and regain their correct natural shape and structure. Persevere.

There seems to be so much to do for me to find my Middle Path. What is the simple answer to this?

To get you up and running, I would suggest you spend a week just becoming conscious of keeping your head upright, with crown pointing up and chin pulled in gently (not stiffly). You should retain this sense of lifting while sitting, standing and walking; you will experience the gradual opening of your torso. Then spend a few days linking the head-lifting to chest-lifting: for example as you lift the crown of the head, feel it pull up the centre of the chest. The goal thereafter is to make that become natural each time you do it. Once you are past this stage, release the pelvis by circling, swinging and twisting it to make it move, as the Chinese say, "Like a free-spinning wheel." After this, bend and straighten your knees in both weight-bearing and non-weight-bearing postures (e.g. standing or squatting; and sitting, lying down or standing on one leg respectively) as frequently as possible to try to recover their full range of movement. That's it in a nutshell.

The statistics for people falling over and injuring themselves are frightening. What is the main cause of this and how can someone like me, advanced in years, avoid it?

As you get older your structural soft tissues (muscles, tendons and ligaments) start to weaken, shrink and lose their structural integrity. This results in loss of flexibility in the joints and in the body as a whole. The joints compress and limit movement, which is the first major culprit in causing falls; the second is loss of gravitational alignment and the third, loss of proprioception. This equates to stiffness, physical balance and inner sense of balance, explained as follows:

STIFFNESS: A stiff standing body will topple over, even with a slight push and especially so when turning to change direction. The waist usually swivels to point in the direction you intend to go, which helps you remain balanced as you step out. What happens in a stiff body is that the waist fails to turn enough and you end up tripping over yourself. Remedy? Stand in Stand Still Posture as shown in Chapter 5. Adjust and relax your posture from head to toe, utilising the breathing to assist the process. Lower the body into the Upright Squat (see Chapter 6), then circle, swivel and swing the waist and pelvis. Follow this by returning to Stand Still Posture with stretching, flexing and twisting and turning of the spinal column. (Details of how to do this safely can be found in Chapters 2, 3 and 6.)

PHYSICAL BALANCE: This is where gravity moves outside your joints, making you unconsciously unstable. Gravity is the instigator in this case. Remedy? Stand for a while in Stand Still Posture, then move your body in the 1 to 4 method shown in Chapter 6. This will help reposition gravity at the centre of the joints.

INNER SENSE OF BALANCE: The combination of stiffness and lack of quality in the full range motion of the body shuts your inner sensors down, leaving your brain confused as to where your body is in space at any given moment. Remedy? Develop your inner senses by standing quietly in Stand Still Posture and breathe slowly and deeply through the nose, placing your mind on your centre of gravity, one inch below your navel. This will open your awareness of the whole body.

How would the Middle Path help my frozen shoulder?
A frozen shoulder responds well to the subtle shoulder and chest movements of Tai Chi and Qigong. The four key locations in the upper body influencing the shoulder are:

Chest (centre of sternum); head (crown pointing up); armpits (open in varying degrees, but never fully closed); and elbows (always off the body). The Middle Path is where you should locate all four of the above for the shoulders to relocate to their natural centre. Apply the directions of the Classics, then roll the shoulders forward and backward eight times each way while lifting and lowering the chest centre. Do this a few times every day and it should have the desired effect.

4

The Qi of Breathing –
For General Health and Respiratory Disorders

The first in-breath = Yang
The last out-breath = Yin
All that goes between = Tai Chi
— *PTN*

Breathing (Huxi) is a grossly underutilized force available to all creatures on this earth. It is only we humans, though, who, uniquely, are able to intelligently tap in to this limitless resource. The ancient Chinese medical and Daoist practitioners were observers and through their research, Qigong gained a whole breathing methodology. In this chapter, we will examine the common errors people fall into with their breathing and look at the various ways the breath can heal and enhance power.

In the mind of the ancient Chinese, respiration was regarded as *the* most important bodily function. They believed it to be the primary source of human Qi (life force) and that it could influence emotions, bolster the Shen (Living Spirit) and provide them with essential energy. And it was no doubt this belief that heralded the development of Huxi Qigong, which in the context of breathing means "The Acquired Skill of Whole Body Breathing." This is meant, over time and with diligent practice, to enhance the quality of the individual's breathing to such a point that health is bolstered and in some cases spiritual enlightenment is achieved.

If Qi is Air and Air is life,
Then nurture, draw and live.
— *PTN*

Researchers in China, at the National Scientific Research Society on Qigong, have made the following observations on the beneficial effects of Qigong practice:

> *"A Qigong practitioner's oxygen consumption in a sitting or lying posture decreases by 30 per cent after performing the exercises. Metabolism of energy also decreases by 20 per cent, as does the frequency of respiration."*

These changes, the researchers asserted, indicate that the practitioner is in a state of "low energy consumption", which can save energy and help build up physique to overcome disease.

Negative Influences on Breathing

Posture

Posture and breathing are intrinsically linked; this is something you can test for yourself with these examples. They are best practised standing, but can also be done while sitting. *Note:* all breathing is in and out through the nose.

- **The Head** – Tilt your head forward with the chin tucked in and take a good in-breath through the nose, sensing how it feels as it goes down through your torso. Compare by then doing it with the head lifted up and slightly tilted back and take another in-breath; you should notice a difference.

- **The Shoulders** – Breathe in as you close both armpits, with the inside of the arms touching the sides of the torso. Now do the same with the armpits open. See and feel how your chest cavity expands more due to this subtle and simple change.

- **The Elbows** – Straighten the arms to the point where your elbows are locked straight. Take a deep in-breath and pay attention to your lower chest and midriff (diaphragm); you will notice it feels tight. Now bend the arms and point the tips of the elbows out and away from the sides of your body. Breathe in and compare.

- **The Hands** – Clench your fists tightly and breathe in. Now do the same with open fingers and palms and compare.

- **The Arms** – Fold the arms across the chest. Breathe in and pay attention to how your midriff and chest cavity feel. Now, unfold the arms and keep the armpits open and compare the feelings.

- **The Chest** – Hollow the chest so it's concave and hold it fixed in that position while you breathe in. Then do the same while raising the chest excessively (so it's convex) and breathe in. Compare the feelings. Now let the chest fall back to the middle and breathe in again. Notice how it feels.

- **The Midriff** – Fold the midriff by holding your pelvis forward and dropping your chest and breathe in. Now compare by lifting the chest and allowing your pelvis to tilt naturally (slightly down at the front).

- **The Pelvis** – Swing your coccyx back and out, which has the effect of tilting your pelvis down at the front, hold it still then breathe in. Then tilt your coccyx under, which tilts the front of the pelvis up and hold. Breathe in. Now allow the pelvis to swing naturally back to the middle and breathe in again. Compare how these three positions feel.

- **The Knees** – Pull your knees back until they are locked straight, touching the ligament wall, and hold. Breathe in. Now compare with allowing the knees to slide forward to an upright middling position and breathing in again.

Environment

In addition to posture, factors such as smoking, air pollution and the Feng Shui of the environment directly affect the quality of your respiration. Smoking needs no elaboration and air pollution speaks for itself. Feng Shui – which means Wind (air that is moving) and Water – considers climatic and environmental conditions that you can be exposed to in your everyday life. For example, if you live on the side of a hill that receives little or no sunshine and so the environment has excessive damp and cold, you are likely to suffer from more chest complaints and arthritis than someone who lives on the side of the hill bathed in sun.

Stress and Anxiety

The multitude of stresses we are exposed to in our daily lives, some without us even realizing, become locked into the body. They create tightening of the diaphragm, chest cavity, abdominal cavity and spinae erector muscles, all essential players in healthy respiration. Stress restricts the natural free-flowing action of the muscle fibres and replaces it with rigidity and stiffness, damaging not only the breathing but also other essential physiological functions. Abdominal breathing can stimulate the vagus nerve, a central stem of the parasympathetic nervous system, which runs through the abdomen, chest and up to the brainstem.

Dr James S. Gorden, founder and director of the Centre for Mind–Body Medicine in Washington D. C., highlights the importance of correct breathing to combat stress: "When you confine your breath to your chest (here he means 'High Chest Breathing', usually caused by mouth-breathing) instead of using your diaphragm (which is linked to the preferred 'Nose-Breathing' method) you increase anxiety." He goes on to state: "The key to 'chilling out' lies in calming your sympathetic nervous system (your body's fight or flight engine, which releases adrenalin and stress hormones such as cortisol) and triggering your parasympathetic nervous system, which controls your rest and digestive functions (the ability to relax and digest your food without the irritation and potential complications caused by indigestion) and helps your muscles and mind unwind."

Clothing

Tight-fitting clothing impacts on the quality of your breathing. Wearing a belt or underwear too tight round the waist; a shirt that's too tight round the chest; or a jacket worn too tight across the shoulders; or carrying a backpack with a tight chest strap – all of these things influence and can impede the ebb and flow of air in and out of the lungs.

Method

How you breathe has the single biggest impact on your health. We are not shown how to breathe when we are children, because in our early lives we do it correctly; but as we age, bad habits kick in and the seeds are planted for future health problems. The following sections cover: where to, when to, how to and how not to breathe and should, in my opinion, be taught to children from the age of eight and upwards as a matter of course.

When and Where to Practise

When

According to the ancient Daoist physicians, the period between midnight and midday is defined as "Seng Qi", "the Time of the Living Breath", which is when the air is being replenished and recharged with "Healthy Qi". In particular, we should participate in refreshing breathing exercises between 5:00 and 7:00 a.m., which is when we usually wake up with our bodies revived to face the new day. This combination of our body energy (Ren Qi) and revitalized morning air (Chen Qi) provides the best possible tonic for our respiratory mechanisms and our health generally.

Where

Choosing the right location was very important to the ancient Chinese practitioners. They understood how location can alter the quality of the air we breathe; for example, you clearly would not practise your breathing exercises standing next to a chemical factory, but standing on a pollutant-free coastline or on the slopes of a mountain would be ideal.

The ancients devised a science, mentioned briefly above, for this understanding of the link between topography and good and bad energy and its effects on human health and prosperity – they named it Feng Shui (Wind and Water). To find the best location to train your breathing, simply seek fresh air. In China it is not uncommon for people to travel some distance from their home in the morning, just to "Take in the Air".

How to and Not to Breathe

The first thing to talk about is the shocking lack of understanding and appreciation of the amazing force that is breathing. During our early years of life we are blessed with perfect posture, perfect breathing and perfect body-mechanics, which together are the essential ingredients necessary for a long and healthy life. These favourable conditions remain untainted until we reach the "Age of Change" (between seven and eight years). This is when the open-eyed innocence of the child transforms into self-awareness and self-consciousness, complemented by parental and authoritarian demands on performance. The result of this is distraction and stress – distraction from living and moving in the free-spirited way the child has enjoyed since birth and stress that throws the mind, body and spirit out of balance. These stresses plus the postural changes that take place as children get older, affect the breathing mechanics and cause them to start to lose their naturalness.

"To live is to breathe."
— *DAOIST SAYING*

The above refers to children without specific respiratory problems. For more on the conditions asthma and COPD (chronic obstructive pulmonary disease) see Chapter 9.

Nose or Mouth?

This is probably *the* most asked question by a totally confused public, who have consistently been given conflicting information on this vital aspect of breathing.

A very good reason to avoid mouth-breathing as your normal regular pattern is the gas nitric oxide. This gas is made by your sinus and mucous membranes and although it is only produced in small amounts, when inhaled into the lungs it significantly enhances their capacity to absorb oxygen (oxygen respiration increases by between 10 and 25%). Nitric oxide is also lethal to any bacteria or viruses that enter the lungs. Mouth-breathing does not produce this friendly gas.

A quick way to feel the difference between nose- and mouth-breathing is to test and compare which of the two has the most calming effect on you. Take a deep breath in through your mouth and breathe out slowly through the mouth – pay attention to its effects on your body and mind. Now do the same with the nose. Nose wins, no contest. Remember the method – it is the out-breath that calms; the in-breath is there to refresh and draw the bow of power. This does not mean you should never breathe through the mouth – nature sometimes guides us to when we exert ourselves: for example when we stride up a hill. Within only a couple of minutes your mouth will drop open to support the struggling nose that is failing to cope with the oxygen demands your body is placing on it. Mouth yawning is part of nature; therefore do not suppress a yawn when the urge arises. When you are bone tired at the end of a hectic day, your body and especially your brain may need a quick fix of oxygen. Your mouth, therefore, is perfectly placed to gulp in the copious amounts required to balance the body.

Worth remembering is that exhaling fully and healthily is just as important as healthy inhalation, because when the lungs cannot exhale and expel enough carbon dioxide, a toxic build-up occurs that is damaging to all the cells of the body.

Something as simple as adopting nose-breathing can alter the internal physiological state of the human body. Clinical studies show that the "Deep Inhalation" (this is usually practised instead of normal breathing) of Medical Qigong breathing therapy increases the stimulation of the sympathetic nervous system, causes blood vessels to contract – which raises blood pressure – and increases the pulse rate. Conversely, the "Enhanced Exhalation" of Qigong breathing therapy has the opposite effect: it stimulates the parasympathetic nervous system, dilates the blood vessels, lowers the blood pressure and decreases the pulse rate.

Inhalation creates a Yang-boosting effect on the internal circuitry (fluid and electric); in contrast exhalation creates a Yin-calming effect on the same circuitry. Chinese researchers have also found that, when both are used correctly, breathing can penetrate much deeper into the body and stimulate much deeper levels than has previously been thought possible, even to the level of keeping the walls of the blood vessels soft and flexible.

> *"I still get frustrated over Western medicine's failure to grasp the nettle of the powerful therapeutic effects breathing therapy can have on so many clinical conditions. Hopefully with the results of the clinical research currently being made public globally, this will change."*
> — *PERSONAL OBSERVATION*

Huxi Qigong

This is probably *the* most beneficial and therapeutic breathing training method that has ever been devised. It targets all the key zones that need to be activated for healthy respiration: the abdomen, the midriff (diaphragm), the thoracic chest cavity and the respiratory airways (larynx, trachea, the bronchi).

1. Resting Exhale Posture:

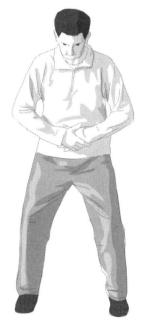

FIGURE 12: Exhale Posture

You will note how the whole length of the spine is at rest (including the head and neck) in a bowed-forward position. This creates the perfect shape for exhalation (through the nose) and at the same time relaxes all the body's soft tissues, which makes the naturally following inhalation more deep and healthy.

2. Abdomen Breathing Posture:

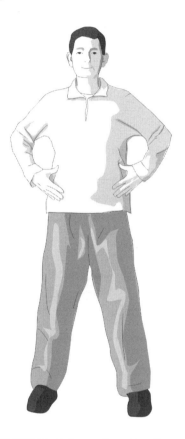

FIGURE 13: Abdomen Breathing Posture

While inhaling, straighten the legs and gently pull back the knees to project the spine upwards and outwards; this opens the abdominal and chest cavities and clears the airways. Slide the palms out and sideways until they reach the sides of the waist at the highest point on the pelvis – the bony iliac crest, which you can feel with your fingers. Have your fingertips touching the iliac crest. Now breathe out and return back to Exhale Posture.

3. Diaphragm Breathing Posture:

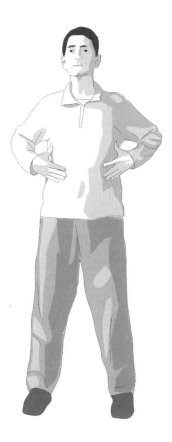

FIGURE 14: Diaphragm Breathing Posture

The midriff is the home of the diaphragm, which is responsible for two thirds of our breathing (the other third taking place in the chest cavity). With the over-lapped palms placed above the navel and fingers spread apart, start to gradually raise the body up from the resting Exhale Posture. At the same time, separate the hands to slide them over the lower ribcage so that you can sense and feel your midriff open and your ribcage expand. Both are vital for diaphragmatic movement. Then return your hands to the centre and slide them back down over the abdomen into Exhale Posture.

4. Upper Chest Cavity Breathing Posture:

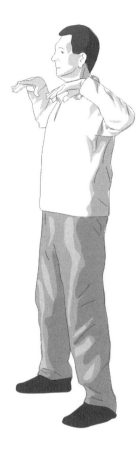

FIGURE 15: Upper Chest Cavity Breathing Posture

Slide the overlapped hands up the centre line of the body as you inhale to the upper chest. Then let them separate so the thumbs can touch the Qi Hui points (Lung One) in front of each shoulder. As the rising hands reach the midriff, the midriff lifts and opens. The same applies as the hands, still together, reach the centre of the upper chest, but when they separate the shoulders raise and roll back to allow the chest cavity to expand fully.

Tai Chi Symbol – Spine Wave Breathing

Also known as "Natural Cleansing Breathing", this exercise links the breathing cycle with the ebb and flow of the rising Yang and descending Yin. This is how we should all train our breathing; it matches the natural opening and closing action of the spinal column, torso and neck with the ebb and flow of the breath. This creates a rising and descending wave action, concentrated in the spine, which links all the key breathing centres that have been explored in Huxi Qigong above. Additionally, Spine Wave breathing fires up the circulation of the cerebral spinal fluid and massages the organs that sit in front of the spine. Start just sitting down on a straight-backed chair, your feet pointing forward, shoulder-width apart with your back straight and head upright.

Spine Wave Breathing, Part One:

1. Place your left palm over the centre of your abdomen and right palm over the centre of your sternum (mid-chest).

2. Now, imagine you are pushing your midriff forward and upward between both hands. You will notice that your neck and head tilt upwards naturally. If you have done this correctly, your hands should be moving apart from each other. Additionally, your mid-spine should be extending inward and upward. This is an in-breath, and should be gradually and gently filtered in through the nose.

3. Next, feel the midriff retreating down and backward, which will bring the hands back towards each other. It will also lower the centre of the chest and the neck/head and bow (like a bow and arrow) the thoracic or mid-spine outwards. This is an out-breath, and should be released effortlessly.

You have just completed the basic cycle; now move on to the rising wave and descending wave breathing cycle.

Spine Wave Breathing, Part Two:

1. With the hands still in place over the abdomen and chest, breathe out and lean a little forward. To create the rising wave, the Inhale sequence should be: Inflate abdomen – Inflate midriff – Inflate chest, in that

HEALTHY AND FIT WITH TAI CHI

order. Start by gently breathing in through the nose and focus your attention on the abdomen. Feel the breath filling the abdominal cavity like air slowly filling a balloon. Then lift the head a little . You will notice that the midriff is now filling with breath. Keep lifting the head and gaze above the distant horizon, while continuing to breathe in. You have completed the inhalation cycle, filling the chest cavity.

2. Part two of the cycle, descending wave, is perhaps surprisingly the same sequence: abdomen – midriff – chest. To perform, start slowly and gently breathing out through the nose as you feel the abdomen deflate, then the midriff and finally the chest. The head will automatically lower itself down to match the out-breath.

With practice, you will develop the essential spine wave breathing connection between the pelvis and the head, an action that harmonizes perfectly with your natural body-mechanics.

Other Remedial Breathing Exercises

Here are a few of many ancient Chinese Qigong therapies for the whole respiratory function. According to the ancient Daoists, they collectively "Appease the sixty-four gods" (in other words, all sixty-four major acupuncture cavities). The principle behind these shapes and body-mechanics is to move in such a way that not only do you open and close the abdominal and chest cavities, but you also stimulate the major acupuncture points and airways.

The key acupuncture points for breathing stimulation are:

- **Qi Hui points** (Lung One, located at the front base of the shoulder joint).
- **Shan Zhong** (Middle Mountain, located in the centre of the chest on the nipple line).
- **Qi Hai** (Sea of Energy, located one inch below the navel).
- **Lougongs** (Labour Places, located at the centres of the palms).

Others are important, but these points are the most responsive to regulating your breathing. When you have mastered the natural opening and closing of these points, you should progress to stimulating them in the body-mechanics of your everyday life (see Chapter 6).

Wave Hands Like Passing Clouds

Also known as "Cloud Hands" and probably the best multi-therapy exercise to come out of China, this routine carries numerous health benefits but is particularly effective for remedying respiratory dysfunction. The major benefit of this routine is how it opens up the right and left thoracic cavities of the chest, in an alternating therapeutic way. The movements involve a large alternating outward circling of the arms, with the palms facing in as you lift and circle the arm and facing out as you complete the circle and descend the arm.

When the palm is facing in you breathe in and when the palm is facing out you breathe out. The performance should reflect the name of the exercise: hand floating slowly and gracefully like passing clouds.

KEY WORDS: Soft, Circular, Floating, Sinking, Transforming, Synchronized and Continual.

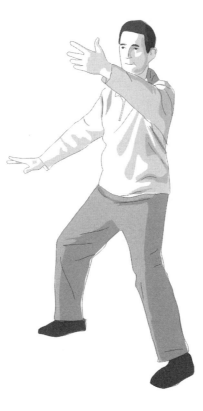

FIGURE 16: Cloud Hands

The Flying Crane

This is where the Chinese saying "The arms are the wings of the lungs" comes into its own. When the arms open and close no higher than the midriff it is also known as "Bellows Breathing": the arms are the handles and the diaphragm/lungs/chest cavity are the bellows, driven by a flexing spine. As the arms are raised above the head as seen in Figure 17, it transforms into the Flying Crane, which reflects the graceful flying action of the white crane – an iconic Chinese bird known for its longevity. As the arms are raised, on the inhalation, the wrists should hang down loose all the way, including when they touch each other above the head. As the arms are lowered, on the exhalation, the hands should gradually be bent at the wrist with the fingertips pointing upwards.

KEY WORDS: Coordinated, Graceful, Beautiful, Soaring, Gliding and Swooping.

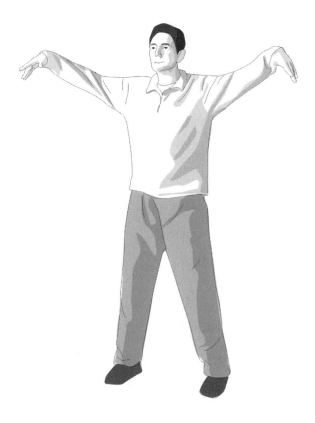

FIGURE 17: Flying Crane

White Crane Stretches its Wings

A beautiful and powerful exercise that acts in a spiral-driven open and closing way, unifying the interaction of shoulders and chest cavity. The arms spread the Qi outwards when opening and direct the Qi inwards when closing. This Qigong exercise alternates the opening and closing of right and left chest cavities, which can help direct healing power to a weakened lung by repeating more arm lifts on that side than on the stronger other half.

KEY WORDS: Separating, Spreading, Stretching, Opening, Closing, Heaven and Earth.

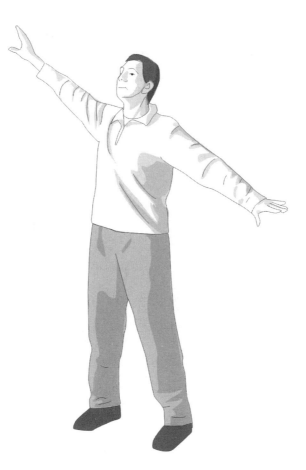

FIGURE 18: White Crane Stretches its Wings

Hands Clasped Behind the Back

This is a very old and established Chinese yogic lung therapy that is known to literally lift and stretch the lung tissue upward through the combination of lifting the head, raising the chest and rolling the shoulders back (see Figure 19 "Open"). The following movement then goes on to relax the lung tissue (see Figure 19 "Close"). This movement is known to Chinese therapists as "Lung Recovery".

1. OPEN   **2. CLOSE**

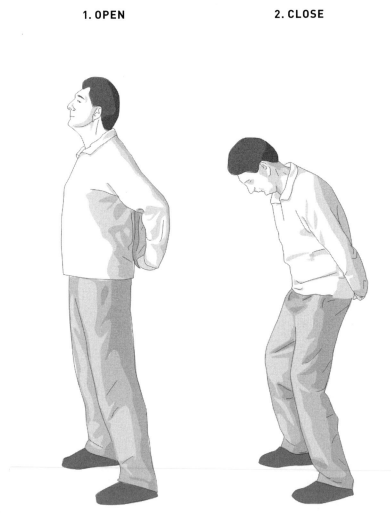

FIGURE 19: Hands Clasped Behind the Back

The title "Hands Clasped Behind the Back" is slightly misleading; it is better to just hold lightly onto the first and second fingers of the other hand. This is called "Holding the Sword Fingers." The reason for this is to create more space to open the armpits and roll the shoulders back and forth.

> *"Qi enters the bones when the abdomen is full."*
> — *I CHING*

Questions and Answers

Why do I find it so difficult to breathe in and out through my nose?
This is because your body has adopted the damaging mouth-breathing method and it is now firmly entrenched in your subconscious actions. You should be patient and allow your body time to return to its natural state of breathing. Start your training with the simple airway breathing method described in Spine Wave Breathing Part One and progress slowly through the routine. Many people breathe tensely because of years of incorrect mouth-breathing and poor posture; when they try to switch to nose-breathing, this is also performed tensely (my own mother demonstrated this perfectly recently). Do not force nose-breathing or breathing in general. Create the right mechanical conditions, relax, persevere and it will reappear naturally.

When I breathe in, I feel I am hitting a wall in my midriff. How do I overcome this?
The "wall" that you talk of is in fact postural stiffness and blockage in the midriff zone between abdomen and chest. Huxi Qigong's midriff breathing is best placed to break down the physical muscular stiffness in the torso. Place your hands on your midriff as described in the exercise and start flexing and extending your spine. Don't focus too much on the breathing at this stage; the practice will soon open up the blockage you are experiencing.

I suffer from COPD and for some strange reason find it difficult to breathe out. What is causing this and how do I rectify it?
Locked-up, fixed head and chest positions tend to deplete a quality out-breath, especially if your fixed position is "elevated chest and head". This according to Chinese Traditional Medicine is when the "Yang Qi is trapped in the upper body." By holding chest and head up you are making it difficult for yourself to breathe out, because this position constantly fixes the airways in the open inhalation position. In contrast to this is the hollow chest, head downward-tilted and fixed (Yin), associated with breathing out.

To remedy the problem, I suggest you stand in Stand Still Posture (see Chapter 5) to work on bowing the spine outwards (towards your back) by dropping the centre of the chest and at the same time, lowering your chin and pulling it in slightly to assist the release of an out-breath (see Figure 12, page 73). Follow this by returning your torso to the undesirable "elevated chest and head" position. Repetitions of this "chest swings up and down" process will loosen the spine and retrain it to centre itself, making it easier to breathe out. You will also notice the quality of your in-breath will have improved.

Would breathing correctly help my recurring indigestion?

Deep diaphragmatic natural breathing is known to assist the whole digestion process, because of how the diaphragm massages the organs as it expands and contracts. Just by returning to this deep but natural state of breathing, your indigestion problem will gradually diminish.

But don't forget, what you eat has an equal effect on the digestive system. The ancient Chinese would say: use the "Metal" element of the lungs to draw the heat of the "Heart's Fires", which means, in simple terms, using deep diaphragm breathing (from the lungs) to cool the rising heat to the heart caused by the indigestion. The same breathing would also be used to draw away the heat in a case of hyperactivity, which is an excessive Yang heart condition.

What would you suggest I do when I feel an impending attack of asthma, and how can I reduce my episodes?

Assuming you have: a) taken your appropriate inhalers and b) notified someone close by that you think you might be experiencing an episode, then the first thing I'd suggest is you make sure you are nose-breathing and not mouth-breathing.

If you do feel the early signs of an attack, place your left hand over the abdomen centre (Qi Hai point) and right hand over the centre of the chest (Shan Zhong point), seek the right fresh-air location (preferably outdoors) and perform Part One of Spine Wave breathing, very softly and gently. As you inhale, when the torso and head lifts visualize all the airways relaxing and opening deep down into the midriff and if possible down into the abdomen. As you exhale, feel the abdomen, midriff and chest muscles settle and relax while you allow the head to gradually tilt down, pulling the chin in (the hands have remained in place throughout the whole inhalation and exhalation cycle).

To lessen the potential for further episodes, embrace the Chinese "Art of Living", encompassing "Healthy Living Form" (see Chapter 6), and practise Tai Chi and Qigong every day (especially Spine Wave Breathing Qigong). All these things will create the protective "Shield" of "Contentment", which is a way of describing the calmness that envelops a person who gains control of their body.

5

The Healing Power Postures – Shapes with Meaning

"In the era of the 'Five Emperor Sages', men dwelt in harmony with nature's laws, knowing well how to remedy sickness and attain a ripe old age."
— *JOHN BLOFELD*

The number of healing power postures contained in the Chinese healing arts is great; in fact too great to cover in this book. The postures I cover here are generally regarded as the "Standards", and cover a broad range of health issues and conditions. They are therefore precious gems, collected from the immensely rich 5,000-year history of Chinese healing, martial and yogic arts. Gems that have been and continue to be an integral part of the Chinese healing culture, they are still nurtured and revered by the present-day masters of these arts.

There are three methods of practice and application: Stationary, Moving and Combined Moving.

1. **Stationary:** The Stationary method involves selecting a chosen posture or postures and holding the body still (Zhan Zhuang), but not perfectly still. There should always remain the natural rise and fall, open and close action driven by the respiratory function. You can use this method for a single targeted benefit: for example, adopting the Earth Posture to calm down an agitated mind. Alternatively, you can enhance the healing power for the same condition by, for example, following Earth Posture with Hold the Centre Posture.

2. **Moving:** The Moving method involves enhancing the natural movement, rhythms and shapes of the chosen posture, to boost the specific benefits it offers. The old Chinese saying "Move Pain" fits perfectly in the context of Moving Healing Power Postures. According to

Traditional Chinese Medicine, pain is the symptom of a blockage and stagnation of Qi, and the first thing the ancient Chinese doctors (known as Fang Shih Prescribers) applied, before administering any pills, medicines or potions, was to move the physical body in such a way as to stimulate Qi circulation through the centre of the blockage zone. Clearing the blockage and replacing it with flowing healthy Qi would resolve most of the conditions that were presented to them.

3. **Combined Moving:** Finally, the Combined Moving method involves performing two or more postures in a flowing and repetitive interacting sequence. I look in more detail at moving combinations of postures, and their ability to target more than one health problem, in Chapter 7. This is known as choreographed combination training and is designed either to stimulate the whole body or target a specific location/condition.

"Without proper motion the body will weaken."
— *TRADITIONAL CHINESE MEDICINE*

The most important thing to understand, whichever of the above methods you choose, is that the basic shapes should be performed as accurately as possible, which is why it is always wise to have the postures checked by a qualified Tai Chi or Qigong instructor. Another important factor in the performance of these postures is summed up thus:

"Energize the shapes, don't just make the shapes."
— *TAI CHI MAXIM*

Anyone can copy the shapes, but this is analogous to looking at a soulless reproduction of an original Rembrandt painting. When performing a healing power posture, you should infuse it with your Shen; by doing so it becomes your own personalized original. The shapes therefore should be full of Qi and spirit, not just technically correct. Inwardly, you can feel how the energized shapes reveal the meaning, usage and application of the Qi, which why these postures are so versatile in their health benefits.

Stand Still Posture
Zhan Zai Yuan Shih

FOR: circulatory conditions (hyper and hypotension), arthritis, central balance, regulating breathing, posture, stress and the energy body.

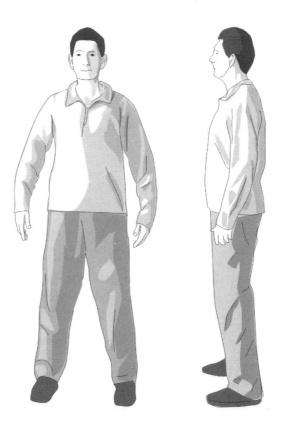

FIGURE 20: Stand Still Posture

According to the ancient Chinese masters: "Whenever the body comes to rest, it should be held in the Stand Still Posture." This is therefore the most important of them all. It is also the most natural posture and comprises feet shoulder-width apart and pointing forwards; the crown of the head to point directly upwards. Shoulders falling away from the neck and armpits open. Chest centre raised and pointing forwards. Eyes fixed on the horizon. Pelvis level and centred. Knees straight and centred. Gravity now sits centrally in the structural joints, allowing the body to regulate itself, free from the imposed conflict created by a lack of postural knowledge.

> *"Stand Still is the unification of Heaven, Mountain and Earth."*
> — *I CHING*

TO PERFORM: With the feet firmly placed on the "Earth" and the head crown touching the "Heavens", you will become as still and as stable as a "Mountain".

> *"Stand Still serves to help the great person attain success."*
> — *I CHING*

Stand Still Posture serves to free the body, mind and spirit from earthly negative influences that would otherwise hamper the health and prosperity of an individual.

> *"A Real Person makes good their position in the middle between Heaven and Earth."*
> — *I CHING*

A "Real Person" is the same as a "Great Person": someone who has attained enlightenment through tuning in to the Dao in everything they do in their everyday life. By "making good your position in the middle" you are exploring the Middle Path, which is the home of the Dao.

> *"He protects his joints by drawing in his knees."*
> — *I CHING*

Again this amazing ancient manuscript describes a key principle in a few words: how pulling the knees back to the middle helps to protect all the structural joints of the body. Centred straight knees bolster and raise the whole body from below, creating structural alignment. This is essential for protecting the joints from the excessive wear and tear of misaligned gravitational force.

NOTES AND BENEFITS

- For additional information on how to adopt this posture correctly, see the Tai Chi and Qigong Classics in Chapter 2.

- It spreads the powerful forces of gravity evenly through the structural joints, freeing the muscles, tendon and ligaments to do their job, which is to create equilibrium, support circulation and enable the natural mechanics of body-motion. Arthritis sufferers in particular will find this posture to be of help, as it evens the load on all the structural joints: spine, pelvis, hips, knees and ankles.
- This is the one and only posture that can be said to benefit any and all conditions that afflict the human form. It is the Middle Path Posture, where the forces of nature operate freely and unhindered, thus keeping the body, mind and spirit healthy.
- It works on the circulation; the openness it creates takes the kinks out of the "hosepipes" (blood vessels) and by doing so, regulates the blood pressure.
- The diaphragm is released from the midriff's vice-like grip (this especially affects people with an Excess Yin posture) and the chest cavity is centred to expand and contract equally and naturally.
- Standing this way acts like a tonic on the central nervous system, allowing it to circulate its electrically charged messages throughout the entire body. This has benefits for people with conditions including cancer, Parkinson's disease and multiple sclerosis.
- When standing still in this posture, let the Dao assist by allowing a gentle rocking motion to manifest, driven by your breaths in and out. This will then calm the central nervous system and help to lower stress levels.

Earth Posture
Jeidi Shih

FOR: prevention of falls, controlling Parkinson's disease tremor, controlling stress, asthma, hypertension, cancer and anxiety.

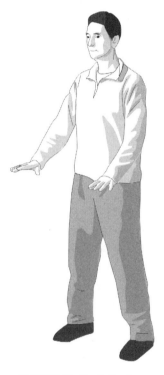

FIGURE 21: Earth Posture

The powerful and impressive Earth Posture stands like a tree with deep roots, which explains why it is called the "Great Stabilizer". This simple to perform body-shape offers more than just physical stability; it anchors the mind and spirit into the bargain.

> *"It represents the end of the cycle and all that is quiet, stable,*
> *earthed and the completion of an outward breath."*
> — *I CHING*

TO PERFORM: stand as in Stand Still Posture, but with the hands (palms facing down) held out a little wider than the hips, as if resting on an imaginary piano keyboard. The best way to experience its power is to combine it with Heaven Posture: start with the hands raised to heaven (see Figure 22) and then lower them down, perfectly synchronized with each other, into Earth Posture.

Breathing Note: With the inhalation complete at the apex of the posture, slowly lower the arms while breathing out through the nose and complete the out-breath as the hands arrive in earth position (see Figure 21).

"Stress is an altered state of mind,
Corrected by a corrected state of mind."
— P T N

When an excessive Yin or Yang posture is maintained for a long period of time, it will impact on the individual's state of mind.

NOTES AND BENEFITS

- People with conditions such as Parkinson's disease will find this posture helps stabilize tremors in the limbs. According to Chinese Traditional Medicine, pain and uncontrolled shaking are a sign of blockage and therefore, to alleviate the blockage you must first physically move and shape the body to encourage the Qi to achieve maximum flow. The Chinese way of increasing the flow is to fill the internal reservoirs, then direct the Qi to be sensed in the location of the "Four Gates" (the centre of both palms and feet), where on the exhalation it transforms into "Heavy Qi".
- It calms the mind, physical body and agitated spirit, but must be applied in total unison with a long and natural outward breath, after first breathing in as you perform Heaven Posture.
- When the Qi becomes trapped high in the chest, as seen in many people with heart conditions, it directs the negative, stagnant energy down to the abdomen, where it can be processed, thus taking the pressure of stagnated Qi off the heart.
- Sustained mental stress has been linked to triggering conditions such as asthma, hypertension, cancer and anxiety. Combining Earth with Heaven (see below), especially in a two-posture moving form, can help to control this stress.

Heaven Posture
Tian Shih

FOR: raising the spirit, refreshing the mind, whole-body energizer, respiration and cardiovascular tonic.

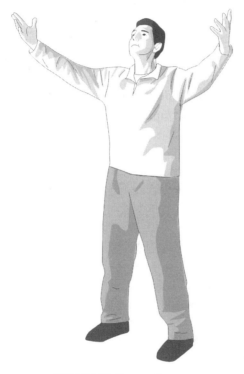

FIGURE 22: Heaven Posture

Heaven Posture, just as powerful as Earth Posture, is performed with the arms, head and Central Channel (Zhong Shen Mai) raised upward to the sky. This according to the ancients allows the spirit (Shen) and life force (Qi) to communicate with the heavenly Qi (Tian Qi).

> *"All that is creative, heaven, the head, the primal power, light-giving, activity, strength of spirit and the apex of the 'in-breath'."*
> — *I CHING*

TO PERFORM: Stand in Stand Still Posture and raise your arms up to the heavens, making the shape of a bowl. The chest and head are lifted up to point to the moon and if performed correctly you should experience an opening of your airways and an uplifting of your spirit.

NOTES AND BENEFITS

- To lift the mood when the spirit is low.
- It refreshes the tired mind by opening up the whole respiratory structure: abdominal and chest cavities, diaphragm, lungs and airways.
- Generally elevates and boosts the Qi throughout the whole body, which has a positive effect on the immune system.
- Its shape maximizes the amount of air the body takes in, which makes for healthy metabolic function.
- The angle the arms are held at, plus the openness of the chest cavity, assist lymph drainage from the arms.
- When combined with Earth Posture in a flowing sequence, it is known to activate the Jinglo (Energy Body) by directing the Qi up and down.

Hold The Centre Posture
Baochi Zhongxin

FOR: centring a scattered mind, centred balance, abdominal health, regulating central nervous system, to re-establish abdominal breathing.

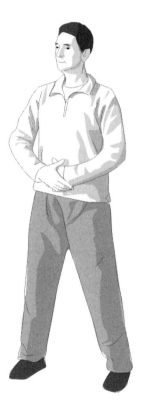

FIGURE 23: Hold the Centre Posture

Placing the hands over the cavity known as the Qi Hai (Sea of Energy) locates the doorway to the centre of gravity for the whole body. The ancient masters also called the Qi Hai the "Mysterious Gate", as it was through this location that according to Daoist tradition "All the mysteries of the universe" could be accessed and it was how they, the masters, communicated with the mind and spirit. By entering this gate and journeying inwards to the absolute centre of the abdomen, you will discover the Zhong Dan Tien (Central Field of Energy). It is here that Qi naturally gravitates to and is stored like a battery, which depending on the individual's lifestyle remains charged or is drained. A charged battery supports all the regular functions of the human physiology and an active balanced lifestyle. A drained battery, however, does not.

TO PERFORM: As Stand Still Posture, except bring the hands to the front of the abdomen with palms facing in and lay them one on top of the other over the Qi Hai point, just below the navel. Men – left hand under right. Women – right under left.

NOTES AND BENEFITS

- The Zhong Dan Tien is the centre of gravity for the whole body and therefore should be regarded as the hub of all actions. This means, in practice, that all physical movements should be guided by and chan-nelled through the centre to create stability, balance and coordination.
- When the hands are placed lightly over the Qi Hai and all the joints are structurally and correctly aligned, the breathing will naturally gravitate to the abdomen centre. The benefits and importance of this for sustained health and natural body functioning cannot be stressed enough. When the breath has returned to its home centre, all of the key operational cogs for healthy therapeutic breathing are in place and coordinating: abdomen centre, midriff – diaphragm centre, chest cavity – Middle Mountain centre and unrestricted airway.
- Centred breathing inside a structurally relaxed, centred body has the additional effect of calming the "Monkey Mind", as the ancients called it. Deep-rooted natural breathing regulates the central nervous system, creating a sense of calmness and clarity of mind, because the "Mon-key" is made to sit quiet.

The Five Bows
Wu Gong

FOR: arthritis, circulation disorders, cancer and immune system.

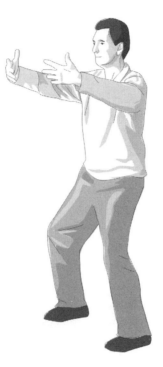

FIGURE 24: Five Bows Posture

TO PERFORM: This is the classic "Squatting While Hugging a Tree" posture, with arms held out at shoulder height and curved as if wrapped around a tree trunk. It is known as the Five Bows because of how it emphasizes the natural curves of the spine and the four limbs, which encourage maximum flow of healing Qi through the meridians. The shapes the upper body make have given it the alternative name of "Upper Body Regulator".

"Seek straightness through a curve."
— *CLASSICS OF WANG CHUNG-YUEH*

To "Seek Straightness" is to be able to find the perfect shape that channels Qi to its maximum; this perfect shape just so happens to be a curve (of the Five Bows).

NOTES AND BENEFITS

- The joints of the skeletal structure are aligned in such a way that they become "buoyant", a favourable condition in which joints are free and open and Qi (in the form of energized blood and synovial fluid) services all the tissues, giving the impression of lightness and buoyancy. With the joints aligned, open and breathing (circulating), arthritis sufferers will notice a drop in their pain and stiffness levels.

"Your body should be so light and nimble that a feather could not land on it without being felt, and a fly could not alight off it without setting it in motion."
— *CLASSICS OF WANG CHUNG-YUEH*

- Lymphoedema is relieved, thanks to the way the pathways are opened between the torso and the four limbs. The spiral action of Tai Chi movement engages the wave-like squeeze and release action of the muscles, which is necessary to motorize the lymphatic fluid.
- The condition frozen shoulder is relieved, especially when working in "combination with Qigong Shoulder Therapy (contact your nearest qualified Tai Chi or Qigong instructor for details). In practice, complete the therapy then perform this posture, holding for a few minutes.
- Those suffering from heart and lung conditions will benefit from the way this posture opens up the connective tissue between the chest cavity and arms. Remember that the ancient Chinese physicians called the arms the wings of the lungs. When the lungs are operating healthily and are free from internal conflict, they support the heart. According to the "Five Elements" principle, the lungs are metal by nature and the heart is fire. When the heart's fires are too strong, the metal element of the lungs (if they are able to perform their respiratory function correctly) draws away this excess heat, which would if left unchecked damage the heart and disturb the emotions.
- The "Bows" of the lower body (legs and pelvis) create perfect conditions for releasing the joints, muscles, tendons and ligaments to operate mechanically in the variety of positions in which they are required to in our everyday physical activities of work and play. The open squatting shape shown in Figure 24 is also known as "Ma Bu" or "Horse Stance", as it creates the impression of sitting on a horse in

a saddle, with both feet in the stirrups. Ma Bu relaxes the buttocks, centres and opens the hip and sacroiliac joints and releases the muscles of the pelvis (front, back, sides and underneath), which allows the pelvis to swing like a pendulum, supporting and coordinating general body-motions, and to self-centre. Collectively all these conditions enhance balance, circulation, the structural alignment of the spine and body-motion in general.

- It can boost the immune system. My first introduction to this special posture occurred approximately thirty years ago when I turned up to train with Master Chu King Hung saddled with a heavy cold. He took one look at me and insisted I stand in the Five Bows Posture while he made me a cup of what he called "special tea". The aches and shivers soon disappeared. He said that the posture would fight off the cold, and he was right. The "special tea", which had what I can only describe as an *unusual* taste, may also have played its part in chasing out the cold.

Push The Mountain Posture
Shan Tui

FOR: anxiety, immune system, Parkinson's, MS, ME and cancer.

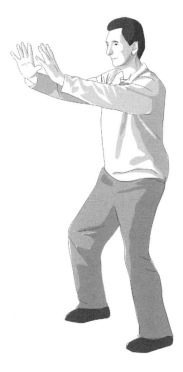

FIGURE 25: Push the Mountain Posture

This is a powerful Yang posture, linked to the element of fire. Of the three directions that a push can be applied in – up, down and horizontally – the horizontal push is the most powerful.

This posture needs some clarification, because despite its name, you do not actually push anything. Instead, all that is required is to make the shape of a push and imagine you are pushing something as immovable as a mountain. This energizes you by leading the Qi with the "Yi" focused mind (see Chapter 2, Tai Chi Classic 5 and Note 2).

TO PERFORM: As Stand Still Posture, but raise the arms up to the tops of the shoulders, wrists floppy with fingers pointing forwards and elbows lifted away from the sides of the body. Elevate the head and chest slightly above the horizon and breathe in. This is the preparation for the push, or the "Seat of Push". Now bend the knees and perform the push as you breathe out creating the shape as shown in Figure 25, with the hands moving straight out from the shoulders.

NOTES AND BENEFITS

- This posture, practised in a moving combination with Seat of Push and Five Bows, forms an excellent circulatory posture-mix that is especially beneficial for the lymphatic circulation.
- Held in stillness for a few minutes daily, this posture will strengthen the mind and body by generating Yang Qi.
- By moving in and out of this posture (flowing between it and Seat of Push), you will realize its physical power in how it creates a very powerful and forceful pushing action. In addition, when applied softly and gently and unified with your breathing, it becomes a powerful heart and lung therapy.
- The inherent physical weakness resulting from conditions such as Parkinson's disease, MS, ME and cancer are countered by this energy-generating posture.

Seat Of Push
Tui De Zuowei

FOR: cardiovascular, respiratory and spinal conditions.

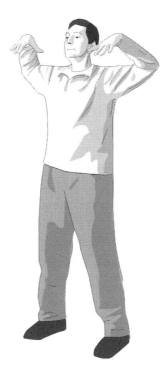

FIGURE 26: Seat of Push

Although this is generally not seen as a full-blown posture, its benefits are such that it is worth including in the healing power posture list. It is worth mentioning that there is an image of this posture on a silk screen excavated by archaeologists in China that dates back to the Han Dynasty (206 BC–AD 220). This posture is known as Seat of Push because it is the foundation of all pushing actions and therefore, not only is it the enabler for a release of Qi, it is also the perfect shape for gathering the Qi.

TO PERFORM: see Push the Mountain Posture above for notes on how to perform Seat of Push.

NOTES AND BENEFITS

- With the hands located, as they are in this posture, in front of the shoulders and the elbows with the chest raised, all the soft tissues that support the chest cavity are opened and stretched. This allows the heart and lungs to function unrestricted, which improves cardiovascular and respiratory function.
- Shoulders influence lung function and general upper body circulation. The upper-body shape made in this posture gently lifts the shoulder girdle up away from the torso. This helps to prevent frozen shoulder and encourages the ribcage to expand and contract fully for healthier respiration.
- There are two ways to perform this posture: martially or for health. Performed as a martial posture it curves (bows) the spine outwards at the back, but performed with health benefits in mind the spine curves inward with the chest raised, as seen in Figure 26. The extension of the spine in Seat of Push and the relaxed releasing of the spine into semi-flexion in Push the Mountain when practised together in moving combination are beneficial for any spinal conditions that stiffen the joints.

Facing Healing Winds
Mian Dui Yuhe Feng

FOR: abdominal conditions, stress and fatigue.

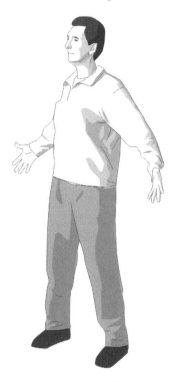

FIGURE 27: Facing Healing Winds Posture

This is a gentle first step in experiencing how the ancients utilized the elements to energize and heal their bodies. They lived much closer to nature than we do in modern times, which enabled them to see and feel the Dao through Feng Shui. Through this ancient Chinese form of geomancy, they could discern where and when positive and negative Qi flowed. Their understanding derived from their observations of how the natural prevailing weather systems (Heaven Qi), interacted with the earth (Earth Qi). The principle is to avoid the locations where negative Qi appears and, instead, locate and embrace the places where positive Qi naturally occurs.

TO PERFORM: The abdomen, chest and head should be slightly raised to expose the Yin parts of the body (which are the most absorbent and most easily soak up external atmospheric Qi). These are: the open palms, the insides of the arms and legs and all front-facing surfaces of the head and torso. The arms are sloping down from the shoulders at 45 degrees with the palms facing outwards.

NOTES AND BENEFITS

- The ancients observed that the weather, including the direction of the wind, affects not just the land but the human body as well. For example, a wind that blows incessantly from the west bends trees towards the east and stunts their branch and leaf growth on the west-facing side. On the other hand, a southerly wind that blows only occasionally will warm a person's bones as they are energized by the sun's rays. The ancients would stand in this posture, facing the wind, to absorb its healthy Qi.
- The whole body soaks up this healthy Qi in this posture, through the lungs and through the pores of the skin all over the body. The palms face the wind to engage the Lougong points in the centre of the hands.
- Although the whole front-facing body is being charged with Qi, with the hands placed out as they are to the sides at waist height, the Qi tends to be concentrated more at the front of the abdomen. This strengthens the flow of healthy Qi through all abdominal organs, alleviating conditions including irritable bowel syndrome, bladder infections and reproductive organ dysfunction.
- The posture also focuses on the midriff and is therefore known to help open the spleen, which is the seat of pent-up emotions.

Balancing Posture
Pingheng Shih

FOR: Parkinson's disease, arthritis, cancer, inner ear conditions, neurological conditions and any other conditions that impair balance.

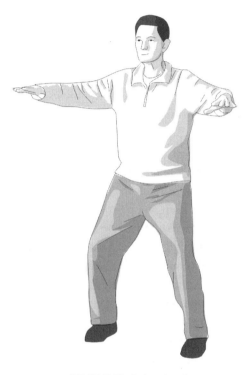

FIGURE 28: Balancing Posture

I first started teaching this to the professional footballers to improve their balance and thus improve their overall performance. It worked so well, I began to think of other ways I could utilize this amazing posture and soon turned my attention to its healing potential. An obvious area is the prevention of falls; this posture is good for conditions including Parkinson's, MS and other neurological disorders. It also works for cancer patients whose balance has been disrupted by chemotherapy.

"Stand as a poised scale and move like a wheel."
— *THE TAI CHI CLASSICS*

TO PERFORM: In order to perform this posture correctly you need to adhere to and adapt your body to the Tai Chi Classics 1 to 4. This will mean you can settle into the required shape without holding stiffness in your joints and muscles.

If you have grasped the feel of the Classics you should first try standing upright with straight legs, knees soft and placed centrally and arms placed "floating", as shown in Figure 28. This will give you a sense of upper-body balance, which you should make sure you are accustomed to before moving on to the next stage as detailed below.

Once you can sense the upper-body balance this creates, you can take it to the next level, which is to encourage the same sensation throughout the whole body. From the straight-leg posture, lower the body down into the "Upright Squat" position also seen in Figure 28. It is essential that you keep your knees soft, light and free of tension. You will become aware of a lightness and buoyancy throughout your whole body; this is the re-energizing of your proprioceptors (your body's neurosensors, which aid balance), and this is your first taste of true balance since you were a small child.

The next stage, while standing in the Upright Squat position, is to turn the waist left and right; start by turning through 45 degrees and gradually increase the turn to 90 degrees. This enhances the flexibility of your lateral spine and torso and trains the waist and head to work in unison, helping to prevent you from falling when you change direction. Turning with a stiff waist and spine and a brain that is being disrupted from sending the message to the feet is a common reason for falls, particularly in the elderly.

NOTES AND BENEFITS

- The frequency of falls in people with Parkinson's is far too common and is due to the stooping and stiffening of their postures. This healing posture combats both of these symptoms.
- For people with arthritis, the structural changes made through performing this posture help take the pressure off the inflamed and stiff joints, which allows the synovial fluids that service the joints of the body to circulate Qi and self-cleanse.

Praying Buddha
Fozu Qidao

FOR: Parkinson's and all conditions affecting mental strength and health.

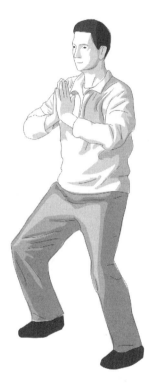

FIGURE 29: Praying Buddha

This is probably the least known in its context as a posture for health; it is much more commonly known in a social context: as the humble bow to show respect. I personally have been using it as a self-control and calming method for people with Parkinson's, especially individuals with the symptom of body twitching. It is also excellent for calming the Monkey Mind, which is usually a symptom of a scattered spirit. In TCM the heart is the residence of the spirit and therefore you need to perform this posture, with its emphasis on the heart region, to "catch the spirit by the tail" and hold it steady.

TO PERFORM: Place the hands together in a praying pose and make sure the palms are only lightly touching each other. Locate them in the centre of the sternum with the fingertips pointing vertically upwards. The elbows should naturally hang down, which will encourage your shoulders to sink. Your core posture should be as in Stand Still Posture and include the gentle rise and fall of the breathing cycle.

NOTES AND BENEFITS

- Visualize an invisible stabilizing pole running through the core of your torso, exiting downward through the feet and upward through the crown of the head. This gives you a feeling of being connected to both heaven and earth, which creates inner stillness.
- For stabilizing tremors or twitching, circle the hands out and up above the head while inhaling, then bring the hands together in front of the forehead. When the palms meet create an audible clap, which will trigger a muscle memory telling the brain it is time to calm the whole body. Then as you exhale, lower the hands down the front of the upper torso, until they arrive at the chest centre.

Questions and Answers

How does Earth Posture help control tremor?
Standing perfectly still in this posture is not enough to control tremor; it requires the support of Heavy Qi. This is created through the supplementary breathing and subtle movements as follows:

> Stand in Earth Posture and breathe in while you lift the hands up – only a few inches – keeping the wrists floppy and relaxed. At the same time open the elbows and raise the chest. The Qi is now slightly elevated to gather at the upper chest and shoulders. Now apply the "4 Down" rule, lowering in sequence: 1. chest, 2. shoulders, 3. elbows and finally 4. wrists. At the end of the sequence you should land perfectly in the Earthing Zone, which only appears towards the end of the lowering sequence when the wrists are gradually settling into the fixed hand position as depicted in Figure 21, on page 91. By naturally and gradually breathing out (through the nose only) as the arms descend, you should sense an inner feeling of heaviness progressing down the arms and filling the hands. This is Heavy Qi – the stabilizer for tremor.

I have a problem with my balance and suffer from a mild form of depression. Which postures should I adopt and how do I apply them?
You need to apply the "Combine and Move" method, which in this case would require repetitions of Balancing and Heaven Postures. Stand in Balancing Posture, turning your waist left and right a few times, then come to rest facing front. Lift up your arms as you inhale and make the shape of Heaven Posture. Hold this posture for three seconds and then lower the arms as you exhale, returning to Balancing Posture. Repeat the whole sequence eight times and you will feel more balanced and emotionally uplifted.

I suffer from COPD and high blood pressure (hypertension); which posture is best for me?
I would suggest you combine Heaven (for respiration) with Earth (for high blood pressure) Posture. Stand for a while in Earth Posture and let your breathing settle

(breathe in and out through the nose) and your body relax. This helps lower the blood pressure. Next, gradually and gently inhale again, synchronizing the breathing with lifting the arms up to perform Heaven Posture. The gradual rising up to heaven opens the abdomen, midriff, chest and airways. Hold for a few seconds, then exhale (still through your nose), gradually returning to Earth Posture. The descending arms and torso assist in the expulsion of carbon dioxide. Repeat the whole sequence four times twice daily, ensuring that your first session is performed in early-morning fresh air. I would also suggest that you practise Tai Chi Form (choreographed sequence) and Tai Chi Walking to supplement the above postures.

I have irritable bowel syndrome and would like to know if these postures would help the condition?
Stand in Hold the Centre Posture and start gradually circling the palms outwards in small circles, then make the circles larger until you are massaging the whole surface area of the abdomen. Do this eight times each way, clockwise and anticlockwise. Inhale as you circle upwards and exhale as you circle downwards; this, combined with the physical massaging, will help balance the large and small intestines. If you wish to calm an overactive bowel, you should massage in circles up the left side, across the navel and down the right side, eight times. If you wish to stimulate a stagnant bowel, you should circle the hands up the right side, across the navel and down the left side, eight times (breathing as previously described). This targets the large intestine. Alternatively, if you find externally massaging the intestines uncomfortable and don't want to physically touch your abdomen, just standing in Hold the Centre Posture while performing deep diaphragm breathing into the abdomen offers the additional benefit of internally massaging all the abdominal organs.

I suffer terribly from stress and anxiety. Which posture is best to help me control both of these conditions?
I would suggest a combination of Stand Still, Heaven, Earth and Hold the Centre Postures. First, you should learn how to just "Stand Still" to bring the body and mind together and create the essential platform from where you will be able to gain the best results from the others. Once you have settled into Stand Still, move on to Hold the Centre until you settle again. Move between them in the sequence Hold the Centre; Stand Still; Heaven; Earth; Stand Still; Hold the Centre. The postures should be stitched together as seamlessly as you can, keeping all movements soft, silky and rounded (no locked straight, stiff limbs or spine). Remember the postures should be fuelled and driven by the breath as discussed in Chapter 4.

6

Healthy Living Form – Natural Body-Mechanics in Everyday Life

*"In a great hurry, he misses his gate and fails
to enter his own house.
To enter the 'Centre Court' of his house, he must conduct
his life in accordance with the 'Mean'."*

— *I CHING*

The Living Form relates to the physical human body in how it must be structured and centred in stillness and motion, throughout every moment of a person's life. According to the *I Ching*, when someone is in a *"great hurry"* their mind is not clear and therefore they cannot see *"the gate to their house"* (errors within themselves). By conducting your life *"in accordance with the Mean"* (the Middle Way), the *"Centre Court"* (a stable home for the spirit) is established. The life force (Qi) and Living Spirit (Shen) unite (in the Centre Court) to guide the body to move correctly and healthily in everyday life. This is a Living Form.

Another way of describing this desired condition is when the Qi of the solid structure is in tune with the Middle Path of the Dao (gravity + universal energy). This centres and opens the body's energy core, known in ancient China as the Tai Zhong Mai (Central Channel), which releases the Shen to shine its light throughout the whole body.

The Chinese have within their culture a maxim for living called "The Art of Living". It entails creating a lifestyle that makes you as healthy as you can be, for as long as you can be. It also involves becoming contented in life, with a peaceful mind; the idea is that if all these elements are in place it becomes possible to achieve the ultimate goal: to die healthy.

Healthy Living Form is the physical element of the Art of Living and, in my opinion, *the* most important if we are going to achieve the end goal and die healthy.

There are two very important ancient Chinese maxims, both of which convey a simple and yet profound message.

"Pain Means Blockage"

Imagine all the body's hard and soft engineering components and internal circulatory systems, including the neurological system, as a multitude of flowing streams of energy that at all costs must remain open and unobstructed. The physiology of the human body has natural shape and form and when the shapes are compromised through poor posture, or physical damage, the energy particles flowing through and around the cells become trapped, like a kink in a hose-pipe, and pain ensues. Pain is nature's way of letting us know that something is blocked and not receiving a healthy supply of Qi. The body is no longer at ease: therefore, a condition of "Disease" arises.

"Move Pain"

This is a very important message, and yet we in modern times still have very little understanding of it. Our usual or "programmed response" to pain is: "It hurts when I move it – therefore I won't move it!" The classic example of this is cracked ribs; until recent times the prescribed treatment for them was to strap the ribs like a medical corset, with tight bandaging, and insist on the patient resting.

The only thing this achieved was to restrict the natural mechanics of the chest cavity, stagnate the vital circulation of healthy healing blood to the damaged tissues, increase the likelihood of lung conditions like pleurisy and generally stiffen the spinal column. Nowadays, people with broken ribs are (thankfully) told to combine rest and movement, supplemented by painkillers as and when required, with no bandaging. So the message is if you have any pain, anywhere in the body, don't sit on it, "Move it!"

"Motion is life."
— *HIPPOCRATES,* Greek physician 460 –377 BC

Essential Living Form Structures

Before introducing the individual Living Form movements, it is essential to explore the natural mechanics of the body's joints: feet, knees, hips, pelvis, spine, shoulders and elbows. This entails looking at the operational ROM (range of movement) of the body's motor components. If any of these components are failing to operate optimally, it can cause a chain-like reaction that negatively affects all the others. Below I highlight what these components offer us and provide guidance on how to keep them operating in a healthy way.

The Feet

> *"The foundation of the whole body.*
> *The 'Point of Contact' with the earth.*
> *The balance 'Sensors'.*
> *The motion originators.*
> *The structural stabilizers.*
> *The circulation providers."*
>
> — *PTN*

To keep the feet operating healthily you must not neglect them; they are there to be walked on. They rely on you putting your full body weight down through them to stay tough, strong and reliable. Public enemy number one for your feet are shoes and should be viewed as a necessary evil, to be worn outside on the streets, or to protect the feet in rugged terrain. At all other times, you should walk with bare feet; this exercises all the complicated hard and soft tissues that make the feet the engineering marvels they are. Here are two special feet therapy exercises:

Rocking From Heels to Toes
This should be accompanied by lifting and lowering the centre of the chest. You will be surprised to discover how the chest and heels communicate intimately in this way. Breathe in as you lift the heels and breathe out as you lower them. Practise as often as you like. This benefits the circulation in the feet, legs and spine and activates your proprioception (sense of balance).

Circling Around the Perimeter of the Feet
As above except that, instead of rocking in a straight line from heel to toes, you roll around the outside edges of the feet while again lifting and lowering the chest and breathing in the same way.

The Knees

"The centre of the legs.
The centre of leg motion.
The power accelerators for the whole body.
The power decelerators for the whole body.
The body's shock absorbers.
The foundation of the hips.
The governors of the hips.
The leg circulators.
The posture influencers."

— P T N

To keep these vital joints operationally healthy, you need to regularly flex and straighten them fully. This means bending them to their full capacity of 140 degrees, so that the back of the calf muscle presses up against the hamstrings and straightening them to the point where the thigh and lower leg are aligned perpendicularly with each other. This exercise should be carried out both when the legs are loaded (when you are standing and squatting) and when they are not loaded (lying on the back with no weight on the legs).

Loaded Knee Exercise
Stand in Stand Still Posture, then gradually bend into a full squat with the hands placed on the knees. At the same time lift the heels off the ground and keep the head upright, spine straight and eyes looking directly forward. Next, while remaining in a fully squatting position, lower the heels while inclining the torso forward. As the heels touch the ground, push down through them to straighten the body up to perform Extended Upright Posture as seen in Figure 30, page 119 (pull both knees gently back to engage with the ligament wall). Finally, allow the knees to relax forward to locate the knee Middle Path centre, which returns you to Stand Still Posture. *Note of caution:* This should be first attempted under the supervision of a qualified exercise instructor.

Non-loaded Knee Exercise
Lie on your back with legs straight, then lift and bend one knee. As you inhale, grasp the knee with one hand and the shin with the other and pull the knee up towards the chest while pointing the toes. To straighten the leg release the hands, placing them on the floor at the sides of the body, and as you exhale straighten the leg while pushing through the heel.

The Pelvis

"The centre of our universe.
The foundation of the spine.
The centre of motion.
The torso waterwheel.
The centre of the breath.
The centre of gravity.
The centre of human reproduction.
The centre of pleasure.
The centre of power.
The centre of energy.
The home of the 'Mysterious Gate'."
— PTN

The pelvis gets a mention in most of the chapters of this book, because it is vital to our health and body function. As you can see from the above verse, take the pelvis out of the equation and life would be miserable for the body, mind and spirit; it influences all three.

To Loosen and Free a Frozen Pelvic Girdle
Stand in Stand Still Posture with knees straight but relaxed and move the waist around in small, then medium, then large circles. Perform this twelve times in each direction. Keep the head steady and upright in the middle while doing so. Now, do the same while holding Upright Squat Posture (see Figure 30, page 119). Another exercise to try is what I call the "Chubby Checker Twist", which the ancients called the "Free Spinning Wheel". It should be performed in exactly the same way as the famous dance, but with the feet fixed not swivelling. The swivelling should come only from the waist and it should be performed much more slowly than the dance. This releases the large muscles that influence and support the pelvic girdle and loosens a stiff lumbar spine.

The Spine

"The conduit for the spinal cord.
The Jade Pillar.
The torso regulator.
The foundation of the head.
The great shock absorber.
The centre of health.

The governor of the four limbs.
The storage vessel of power.
The major 'Bow' of the 'Five Bows'."
— P T N

The spine was in ancient times called the "Jade Pillar"; named after a precious stone that to the Chinese was so important only the Jade Emperor himself could use it in his title. This is how special the Chinese believed this vertical chain of vertebral joints to be; they knew it was, as they called it, the "Conduit of Life". This precious structure needs to be maintained in good working order by regularly extending, flexing, twisting and tilting it.

The most important thing we can do to show the "Emperor" spine our respect, in addition to the above recommendations, is to ensure that our head sits centrally at its top at all times, whether we are sitting, lying, standing or walking.

The Elbows

"The centre of the arms.
The governors of the shoulders.
The shock absorbers for the shoulders.
The shock absorbers for the neck.
The facilitators for the breath.
The directors of Qi.
The arm's power accelerators."
— P T N

The elbows are probably *the* most misunderstood parts of the engineered human body. They are, to most Western minds, those bendy pointy things that keep getting in the way and cause pain after too much golf, tennis or gardening. As seen in the above verse, though, they are incredibly versatile and provide a wide variety of useful regulating actions. To maintain these hinged marvels we simply need to regularly bend and straighten them (preferably in the unique yet natural "Arm Spiral" Tai Chi technique), with our breathing supporting the action. A quick and easy guide to relieving tennis elbow is to repeat and combine the actions shown previously in the two healing power postures of Seat of Push and Push the Mountain.

The Shoulders

"The upper body regulators.
The root of the arms.
The breathing regulators.
Outer protective bumpers."

— P T N

The shoulders, if kept healthy through being free from tension, free moving and open, will influence all those things listed above. Sadly, most new students to my classes usually have "locked-up" shoulders that demonstrate a very limited range of motion, locked up in one position (usually excessively raised) and contributing little to the harmony of body and breathing.

There is another important principle to understand in the interpretation of Living Form: that of its place in our everyday lives. Human movements are meant without exception to be in tune with nature; this obviously applies not just to your practice of Tai Chi but also to your everyday movements, however mundane they may seem.

"Living Form is Tai Chi in all actions."

The Fundamental 1 to 4 Method for Lowering and Raising the Body

The two fundamental actions of human body-mechanics, raising and lowering the body, are often performed incorrectly, leaving pulled muscles, tendons and ligaments in their wake. When performed incorrectly, energy is wasted and damage is done; however when performed as a living form with correct body-mechanics, the actions become pure therapy. The all too common method of squatting down, which is detrimental, is performed with:

a) The head projecting too far forward.
b) The feet often splayed out, misaligning them with the knees.
c) The pelvis tilted and fixed, creating stress in the sinews as the body is lowered (see Sitting on the Pelvis, Figure 10, page 56).

Another area affected by bending unnaturally and incorrectly is the midriff (home of most of the torso's organs and the diaphragm), which tends to collapse and kink, restricting breathing and organ function. This places great strain on the soft tissues of the lower back and sacrum; to rectify this you should follow the Fundamental 1 to 4 method, which engages all the major flexor and extensor muscles of the body – correctly.

1.	2.	3.	4.
STAND STILL POSTURE	**UPRIGHT SQUAT**	**FULL SQUAT**	**EXTENDED UPRIGHT**

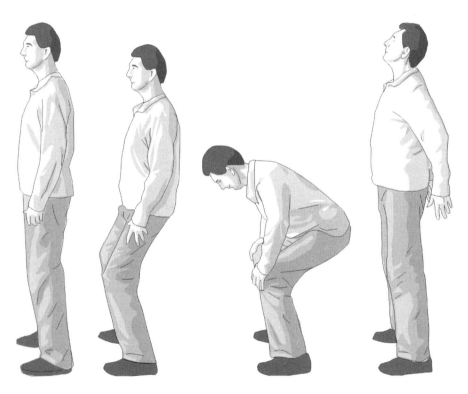

FIGURE 30: 1 to 4 Method

Applying the 1 to 4 Method

When performing this method, it is important to follow the correct, safe sequence of coordinated mechanics: to lower the body move with first the knees, then the pelvis, then the chest and lastly the head. To raise the body back up (stages 3 to 4), follow the same order of movement. Starting from Stand Still Posture, lower the body in the following sequence:

- **Position 1.** Keeping the spine straight, inhale then commence exhaling as you bend into Upright Squat and gently open the knees as if sitting upright in the saddle on a horse (See image 2 above).

- **Position 2.** Continue exhaling as you place both hands on the fronts of the upper thighs and bend the knees a little more, while swinging the pelvis back out of the way. Lower the centre of the chest, without folding or creasing the midriff. Finally, allow the neck joints and head to also lower and focus the eyes on the earth a few inches (10 cm) in front of the toes. At this point the hands will have travelled down the thighs and be firmly placed holding the knees (see image 3).

- **Position 3.** Stretch the whole body gradually up as you inhale, pressing the hands down onto the knees or thighs to assist with moving the chest and head to face up to the moon (see image 4). This Extended Upright Posture creates the perfect shape to exhale and relax the body back into Stand Still Posture.

As always, the breathing should be integrated and synchronized with the movements: breathe out through the nose to relax the soft tissues when performing postures 2 to 3. The out-breath relaxes the supportive soft tissues so that there is no risk of tearing and pulling muscles, tendons and ligaments. *Note:* This method of squatting should be used if you need to bend over to pick up a heavy object, rather than doing so with the knees locked straight.

> *"The reason so many Westerners have*
> *bad backs is because they don't squat."*
> — *MASTER MICHAEL TSE*

Sitting

This is a common action (or more accurately, non-action) that is misunderstood by many and damaging to the body when performed incorrectly. The accumulative effect on the spine and organs of slumping when sitting, categorized in Tai Chi and Qigong as misaligned Yin, is excessive wear and tear on the vertebrae and compression of the organs. Even the actions of lowering the body on to the seat and standing back up are detrimental if these actions are mechanically weak. For example, when lowering the body down to sit, if the body is "dropped" from a height onto the seat instead of being gently lowered in line with gravity, there will be excessive compression of the discs in the spine. Getting up from a seated position is also often performed clumsily, requiring in some cases two (or more) attempts because the feet, knees and head were not aligned correctly. Many people, especially those who are elderly, experience falls when trying to do this.

"When sitting up straight, the spirit of
Vitality remains."
— *P T N*

Living Form Method of Sitting Down in and Getting Up From a Chair

1. **Lowering the Body to Sit:** This should be performed with the back of the legs lightly touching the front edge of the chair seat. Then, by following the guide to squatting down (Numbers 2 and 3 of "Applying the 1 to 4 Method" above), the bottom can be safely lowered on to the surface of the chair. Once seated, lean the torso forward by folding from the hips, making a wedge shape of the spine and backs of the thighs, then slide back, placing the coccyx at the base of the chair-back. Push down with equal pressure on the knees with both hands and gradually stack all the joints of the spine, one on top of the other (including the neck vertebrae), until the torso is held in the same erect position seen in Stand Still Posture.

2. **Getting up from the Chair:** To return to a standing position, slide the bottom forward so you are close to the edge of the seat, place the feet (with the heels aligned vertically to the front edge of the seat) hip width apart with toes pointing forwards. Place the hands on the knees and incline the torso and head forward, locating the chin in line with and centrally between the knees. Then follow the directions described in Number 3 of "Applying the 1 to 4 Method" to rise safely to a standing position. Make sure that you sense the head lifting the rest of the body up as you get up.

Natural Extension and Recoil of the Limbs

This simple, everyday repetitive action is grossly misunderstood and often performed incorrectly. Countless times in the course of our normal daily activities. we use our arms to reach out (extension) and grasp hold of something and return it (recoiling) close to the body. Imagine how much unnecessary wear and tear the joints are subjected to if, as is very often the case, the body-mechanics we use are wanting. Now consider the benefits that might be derived from performing the same action with movements that are positively therapeutic. Suffice to say, the joints of the arms and spine, which absolutely rely on physical motion to stay healthy, will be kept open and breathing, encouraging the maintenance of healthy tissue (cartilage, ligaments and tendons) and circulation (lymph, synovial fluid and blood).

> *"All movements should be natural and in harmony with Gravity and body-motion, to avoid carrying the limbs."*
> — PTN

Living Form Method of Extension

To move the arms the action must commence in the feet (when standing) or in the feet and pelvis (when sitting). It involves a wave and a sequence of movements, which must be performed in the right order. The wave is described below and the sequence of joint-to-joint actions to raise and extend the limbs is as follows:

Feet; knees; hips; sacrum; lumbar spine; Middle Mountain (chest centre); shoulders; elbows; wrists; fingers. See Figure 31.

1. **Standing:** Let's say for example a tin of biscuits is sitting on a shelf at eye level and both hands will be required to perform the task of picking it up and lowering it down on to a waist-height tabletop. Stand in Stand Still Posture, directly facing the tin, slightly bend and slacken the knees and push both feet into the earth. This will create a resultant upward rising wave of force (Jing), which is borrowed from the earth to raise and extend the body and limbs to reach out and grasp the tin.

   The wave must be maintained at a constant rate, through adopting a smooth coordinated joint-to-joint action, free from any pauses or jerkiness and at a frequency that is neither too fast nor too slow. Too fast and muscles will begin to tense and accuracy and control of the limbs will lessen. Too slow and the essential rising power will diffuse, leaving little or no "end power" to perform the task. The breathing should work in perfect harmony throughout this rising action: breathing in starts as the feet push down into the earth and continues as the wave gravitates upwards to the wrists. When the wave arrives at the wrists, the final extension of the hand to touch its intended target should be on an out-breath. *Note:* If performed correctly, lifting the arms should feel effortless.

2. **Sitting:** To raise and extend the limbs in a seated position, it is necessary to move the pelvis forward away from the chair-back, leaving approximately a 50 mm gap. This allows the pelvis to rock back and forth on its base, which in turn releases the spine to flex and create the rising wave, as described in the standing method above. The application and sequence of joint-to-joint action to create the rising wave is thereafter exactly the same as in the standing method.

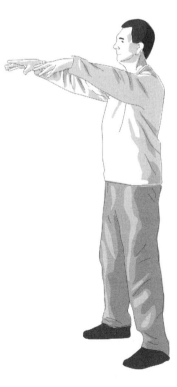

FIGURE 31: Double Limb Extension Posture

Living Form Method of Recoiling

Having extended the limbs through Living Form's total body coordinated movement, the hands have arrived at their destination, the biscuit tin. Now it has to be lowered down on to the tabletop.

To recoil and lower the limbs, initiate the first action at the Middle Mountain (chest centre) by lifting the chest up as you inhale, which will recoil the hands and arms back towards the shoulders. Next, allowing the chest to naturally lower towards the earth as you exhale (and simultaneously lowering the elbows) will sink the shoulders, allowing the body-mechanics to sink the Qi, the arms and the biscuit tin. The biscuit tin will now be lowered to the tabletop on an outward breath and if performed correctly, it should also feel effortless. *Note:* As with the extension method of breathing, the breath should be intimately coordinated with the complete action of lowering the limbs, from beginning to end.

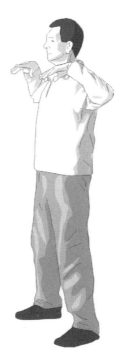

FIGURE 32: Double Limb Recoil Posture

Single Arm Extension and Recoil Method

This method of movement directs the mind and Qi into one side or one limb of the body. It enhances the mobility and motion of the arm in normal everyday activities and, in addition, is a way of stimulating the one side of the body if it has been weakened by, for example, a stroke, Parkinson's Disease, MS or polio. If one side of the body is weaker than the other and the person isn't given treatment or therapy, that side's range of movement tends to decline badly, as does the health of the supporting soft tissues. Hands become claws, elbows are permanently bent, frozen shoulder becomes the norm, the chest cavity is depressed, the spine is bowed and fixed, frozen girdle is established, hips stiffen and knees become permanently bent. The good news is at least some of this can be avoided with the implementation of regular joint-to-joint stimulation.

1. **Single Side Extension Method:** The power mechanics between the feet and the hips are the same as in double hand extension in the "biscuit tin" movement above. However, in order to direct the soft Jing (visible physical moving energy) into one side of the body, the hips must turn to the side as soon as the rising force from the legs reaches them. Turning the hips to the left will "charge" the right side of the body and vice versa. The joint-to-joint spine wave action described in the double hand version applies here too.

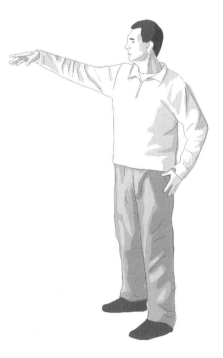

FIGURE 33: Single Side Extension

Remember to set the eyes on a target and imagine soft white light flowing outwards from the fingers to it. This exercise applies whether you are lifting the limb to the level of the waist, chest, shoulder or above head height.

2. **Single Side Recoil Method:** Having fully extended the limb and breathed out, the next step is to return the hips to face front.

   Breathe as you lift the chest and elbow, while drawing the wrist back towards the body (this is the recoil). Then lower the limb and return it to rest at your side, following the sequence of movements described in the double hand recoiling exercise above and breathing out as you do so.

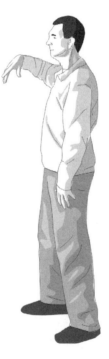

FIGURE 34: Single Side Recoil

"Nature is always in motion, humans should also strengthen themselves without interruption to motion – the body relies on motion to stay healthy."
— *I CHING*

Living Form Fundamentals

Inner Messages

Living Form also means to listen to the body's internal messages, which – if we are tuned in to the natural rhythms of the Dao – tell us when to eat, drink, work, rest, sleep, catnap, sneeze, yawn, cough, cough up, go to the toilet and when to engage in or abstain from lovemaking. Many people find it difficult to take note of these inner impulses, but they are important; they are specifically designed by the Dao to keep the body healthy and regular. The answer is simply to acknowledge that these Dao signals actually do exist and to set up a positive lifestyle that maps perfectly onto the "Internal Dao Clock". In order for us to be able to listen to our inner messages, we must create the conditions for the brain and organs to communicate. The ancients called this "Establishing the wisdom mind".

Restimulation

When our bodies are at rest and paused in stillness, for example sitting watching a movie or on a long-haul flight, stagnation can set in. In health terms this means a noticeable drop in life-giving and sustaining circulation. At the core (Middle Path) of body-motion are the spine and pelvis, which together can, through coordinated flexing and rotation, ward off stagnation. Whether sitting down, standing or lying you should try to send these ripples of stimulation through all the joints, via the pelvis and spine, every twenty minutes. To perform Restimulation you should attempt to gently and slowly move all the body's joints: toes, ankles, knees, hips, pelvis, spine, shoulders, elbows, wrists and fingers in a unified ripple effect. Breathe in as the wave of movement builds and out as the wave settles.

Self-Centring

Many of the everyday physical actions we perform can to varying degrees move the body away from its natural forward facing and upright neutral position, or home centre. A very common postural error is to complete the physical task you have asked of your body without giving any consideration to returning it correctly and naturally back to neutral.

When stretching up, squatting down and twisting left or right, you should allow the natural elastic properties of the muscles and tendons (and to a minor degree the ligaments), to return the relaxed body back to its home centre . Only when you tune in to the Dao and abide by its actions in this way can it say to you: "Hwan Ying Wei Jar!" ("Welcome Home!").

A Healthy Living Diet

Over many years I have observed the changing advice of various "experts" on what we should or should not eat. I have often been dismayed at how many times they contradict themselves. I have always advocated following a healthy, fresh-food Middle Path diet and simply listen to what food our body is requesting and when. But this must not be confused with cravings, which are a testimony to human weakness and can damage body, mind and spirit.

Calorie Burning Form

Try to move your body – deeply and not in a token shallow way – regularly throughout the day. By "deeply" I mean by exercising the larger muscles: thighs, buttocks, chest and back; these are the most effective for fat-burning. Here are some interesting facts to consider: Researchers at the Mayo Clinic in the USA have found that leaner people tend to stand and move more than overweight people in everyday life. Standing, bending, stretching and twisting the muscles burn off fatty cells. The study found that those who lead a more sedentary life and sit for long periods retain 350 more calories each day.

Arthritis Research UK report in their quarterly magazine *Arthritis Today* that for every pound of weight gain (over and above the normal weight for a person's height and age) the physical pressure on the hips is increased by a factor of six. As for the impact carrying extra weight has on the knees, the researchers reported that the knees are subjected to three pounds of added stress for every pound a person gains. Could this be contributing to the increased need for hip and knee replacements in our overweight societies?

The John Hopkins Arthritis Centre in Maryland, USA carried out similar research into what happens to the knee joints during walking in overweight people and discovered that being only ten pounds overweight increases the force on the knee by 30–60 pounds with each step.

Sporadic exercising is as ineffective as sporadic dieting. Consistency is the key, which is exactly what you achieve when you apply yourself to Healthy Living Form.

Tai Chi's Middle Path approach is eminently suitable for regulating body weight due to its integrated body-motion and core coordination methods. Because of this, no areas of the body are allowed to stagnate and build up fatty cells.

Maintaining good core posture helps keep the body open to transport oxygen to the cells and visually, the bulges do not seem so obvious, because an upright torso pulls the stomach and abdominal muscles into better alignment, making you look slimmer even if you are not.

Naturally deep abdominal breathing drives the digestive system to work more efficiently, which converts the fuel of food into more energy and less fat.

How much fat is burned off depends on the ability of the cardiovascular system to deliver enough oxygen to the cells in sufficient time. Physically active people may have up to twice as many capillaries (tiny collateral blood vessels) servicing the muscles than the average less active person.

Note: The more capillaries that are carrying oxygen, the more fat-burning metabolic action takes place. Tai Chi is aerobic by nature.

Experts say that to realize efficient weight loss, it is better to practise a variety of exercises than stick to the same limited regime. Tai Chi has literally hundreds of exercise options.

Tai Chi stimulates the deep transverse abdominal muscles, creating a strong flat tummy and giving extra support to the lower back.

Questions and Answers

How do I 'Move Pain'?

Pain is the body telling us there is a blockage in the normal healthy circulation to the problem area. To move pain does not just mean you moving your limbs; it encompasses massage techniques as well. For example, to speed up the healing process in a case of tennis elbow you can extend and flex the elbow joint and circular-massage the joint, followed by stroking down the arm, over the elbow and out through the hand. This is moving pain.

How do I die healthy?

This phrase may sound contradictory, but there is sense in what the ancient Chinese say. In the Western world we are quick to blame our aches and pains on our age, which is reinforced when you visit the doctor. After examining you he or she announces "It's a bit of arthritis." You say: "What's caused that?" and he or she replies: "It's your age." We then go away simply accepting that this is the future for us now. To die healthy simply means you keep your mind and body as active as you possibly can within sensible bounds – depending on your age and overall condition, of course. The Chinese feel they have achieved this when they pass away with very little prolonged suffering.

Describe the everyday actions I could turn into therapeutic 'Living Form'?

Well, in principle all physical actions are meant to be Living Form. However, there are some that are particularly good because of their mechanics. Vacuuming uses the waist, extension/recoil of the arm and weight transference between front and rear leg. Window-cleaning is great for moving the waist and stimulating the shoulders, and it engages the knees as you move up and down. Wiping down surfaces like worktops is good, and is best performed in a wide Horse Stance, with the body weight slowly transferring from one leg to the other as you wipe the surface by turning your waist.

What is the secret to healthy living?

There is no mystery or secret involved; if you are content, healthy and enjoy an active life, you don't need me to tell you what to do. Many people do find their Middle Path of healthy living unaided and if you were to analyze how they achieved it, each person would have got there with differing actions, likes and dislikes.

Will Healthy Living Form ward off common diseases such as arthritis, heart disease and cancer?
If you are abiding by the doctrine of the Art of Living, which has at its core Healthy Living Form, you are reducing your chances of developing those diseases mentioned and many more, simply by keeping your Qi consistently strong.

7

Middle Path Walking –
Mechanics of Healthy Walking

Along the river bank I stroll
With hands behind my back,
I'm walking slow to breathe the
Air, along the river track.

— *P T N*

It would be inexcusable to write a book on the fundamentals of human health without making reference to the importance of healthy walking. In recent studies many health experts point to Tai Chi and Qigong as being recommended daily exercise methods in the fight against cancer, alongside yoga and walking. In this chapter, I will examine the mechanics of Tai Chi Walking and highlight the hazards of the unfortunate and all too common unhealthy walking methods many people unwittingly adopt.

The first question to consider is why do we walk? We walk simply because we are programmed to, driven by an instinct that dwells within all creatures with legs, implanted in our genes by the Dao. And it is also the Dao that ensures our feet, ankles, knees, hips, spine and shoulder girdle are aligned and engineered in such a way as to capture and centre nature's force (gravity) to motivate the action of walking. We therefore must maintain this joint-to-joint and muscle-to-muscle engineered alignment to walk efficiently and healthily. Unfortunately, many people unwittingly walk in a way that is inefficient and will do nothing positive for their health.

Fundamental Errors in Walking

The most striking thing, to me, is just how many people are unaware of the dangers to their health caused by poor mechanics when walking. The body is engineered to move in such a way that it is self-sustaining and maintaining. The joints, bone shapes, muscles, ligaments and tendons create a body that, when walking as nature intended, can truly be described as poetry in motion. Unfortunately most people unconsciously slip into bad postural habits, which over time interfere with the natural mechanics and rhythms of motion. Walking and posture are inseparable, in good ways and bad. Poor posture directly inhibits the important walking muscles of the pelvis and legs and, through the resultant adverse gravitational forces, the spine, hips, knees and feet suffer excessive wear and tear.

Yin Heel Walkers

This is when the centre of gravity (Middle Path) is allowed to slip back into the heels, creating the effect of ploughing the earth and pounding while walking. With the weight thus firmly embedded in the heels, each time the lead foot is placed down it hits the ground so heavily that it creates a rebound action that travels up through the legs, into the hips, sacrum and spine, damaging the shock-absorbing soft tissues of cartilage and discs. This damage is compounded further by most of the body weight being shifted back into the spine, which creates a heavier than normal working load in those joints. Other considerations:

- The essential Qi becomes trapped in the lower limbs, which weakens the upper body. This manifests as a drawn, pale complexion, weak voice, low spirit and muscle-mass wastage.
- Pain tends to manifest in the rear of the body (spine, sacrum, neck and kidneys).
- Painful calcified spurs on the heel are common.
- Sudden shifting of the gravity line into the toes with full body weight can trigger plantar tendonitis.
- Achilles tendons stiffen and are more likely to rupture when sudden physical loading is applied.
- Calf muscles are overworked and overloaded, leaving them in a persistent state of stiffness.

Yang Tiptoe Walkers

This is caused by a forward-tilted pelvis that throws the abdominal organs out of alignment and the centre of gravity into the balls of the feet instead of the centre of the foot. It is often associated with people who are overweight, but can affect any body type or shape. Visually these people look as the name implies – as though they are tiptoeing over something every time they step forward. These are the opposite to the heel walkers above in that they tend to walk more lightly on the earth, but depending on their weight the walking can still have an adverse impact further up in the body. Other considerations:

- People who "tiptoe" will often complain about pain in the lower back, due to the excessive lumbar curvature it causes.
- The shin muscles are overworked and overloaded, which makes them lose their elastic properties.
- Knee pain is common, due to the excessive loading placed forward from the centre of the knee joint into the kneecap.

Flip–Flop Walkers

This is produced by a Yin slumped posture with limited knee and hip movement. It is also associated with collapsed arches in the foot and generates an erratic stop-start walking action. People with this tendency are closely linked to the heel walkers, but a unique feature is the complete loss of springy tendon action in the feet and ankles. Other considerations in addition to those listed under "Heel Walkers":

- Often complain of pain in and around the ball of the foot, caused by the incessant pounding every time the feet are lowered.
- The erratic stop-start action tends to make the head nod up and down and back and forth (a type of repetitive slow-motion whiplash action), putting unnecessary pressure on the neck vertebrae.
- The knees will also be subjected to the same action that damages the neck, but with the added disadvantage of having nearly all the body weight impacting on the joints.

Toes-Splayed Walkers

Visually this looks as though both feet have fallen out with each other as they endeavour to head off in different directions (see Figure 7, page 35, image on the left). The angle the feet turn outwards can vary from 0 to 45 degrees and the bigger the angle, the more damage will ensue. At its worst this walking style undermines the natural supportive structures (centred joints, ligaments, tendons and muscles) between the feet and the pelvis. The small bones, muscles and connective tissue of the feet give us our connection to earth and therefore our balance. How far the feet move away from straight and healthy alignment corresponds with the level of reduction in the feet's proprioception. Other problems this causes:

- This posture pushes the hip joints back and restricts the hip's range of movement, which increases wear and tear on the back face of the ball-to-socket interface.
- The sacroiliac joints, which join the pelvis to the sacrum, are unnaturally and excessively fixed in the closed position, which radiates stiffness up the spine.
- The lower abdominal muscles are allowed to weaken, which encourages the pelvis to tilt forward. This sends the gravity line towards the front of the body, disturbing the equilibrium.
- The inevitable distortion of the knee mechanics in this posture results in strain, pain and weakness. Knees turning outwards, as directed by the outward-turning feet below them, tend to collapse inwards because gravity still tries to follow a straight line down to the earth.
- There is a noticeable loss of buoyancy, shock absorbency and power in the knees.

Flat-Foot Shuffle Walkers

People with this walking style do not point their toes down when lifting their feet as they should, or bend their ankles when lowering them. In other words, the feet retain one fixed position: parallel to the ground. They can be quickly singled out in a crowd as they are the ones who move with a fixed head height. Hence this is also known as flatline walking. Other considerations:

- Shufflers have stiff ankles and lower leg muscles, which restricts the natural flexing of the ankle joints.
- The circulation of Qi, blood, lymph and synovial fluid (in the joints) becomes stagnant throughout the body, but especially in the lower limbs.
- Ankle and leg proprioception is dramatically reduced, to the point where falls are more likely than not.
- If the feet do not have natural "fall contact" (heel placement) with the ground, the pelvis becomes fixed and stiff, losing its shock-absorbing ability. In addition, the spine is now exposed to damaging forces arising from the action of the flat feet.

Upper-body Errors in Walking

In addition to errors in the mechanics of the feet, many people adopt upper-body actions that only serve to enhance the damage the lower body errors cause. When the head, chest and shoulders are misaligned it also interferes with the natural health-enhancing swinging movements of the arms, as seen below:

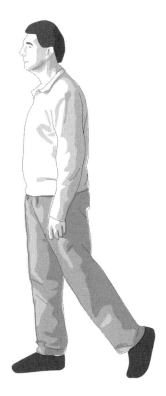

FIGURE 35: Restricted Arm Swing

Tightness in the chest and upper back muscles tends to do the same to the shoulders; this is why many people develop restricted elbow swings instead of healthy shoulder-root swings.

Healthy Walking –Technique

Healthy walking should be effortless, but for many it is difficult simply because walking relies on good posture, which as we have seen is quite uncommon in our Western world. Assuming the previous chapters have corrected your posture, you now need to understand correct and natural technique. To help gather the key components, I have written the following verse, which contains all that is necessary for healthy walking.

ONE STEP

One step to walk with nature
To roll from heel to toe.
One step to swing the hip –
To swing it to and fro.

One step to flex the knee joint
And accelerate along.
One step with kneecaps pointing straight,
To make the knee joint strong.

One step with crown point lifted
And eyes that look ahead.
One step with arm-swung shoulder root,
Swung light and not swung lead.

One step with pelvic twisting
And chest that twists as well.
One step that makes the torso coil,
Together they self-propel.

One step with all these things as one
United in fluid motion.
One step and then another,
The true way for health promotion.

— *PTN*

Three Methods of Tai Chi Walking

1. **Free and Easy Wandering**: In Figure 36, we see a posture where the hands are clasped behind the back: Holding the Sword Fingers. This is when one hand lightly grasps the first and second fingers of the other hand, forming a recycled circuit of Qi through the arms. This posture (in motion) is also described by the ancient Chinese as "Strolling along the riverbank", which means it is to be walked at the same pace as a meandering river.

    The position of the arms opens the chest by gently extending the shoulders outwards, without forcing them back. So now we have open chest, open shoulders and open lungs, which collectively relaxes the whole upper body. This body-shape also exposes the front (Yin) of the torso and helps you absorb the healthy surrounding Qi through the major cavities linked to torso breathing (see Chapter 4). Another observation is the way it is possible to tune the steps in to the rhythm of the breathing, as opposed to the other way round. Each time you step forward to place heel of the leading foot down, you will notice the chest lowering (this is an out-breath).

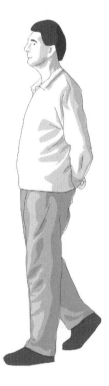

FIGURE 36: Free and Easy Wandering

When the rear foot lifts and pushes off to swing forward, it lifts the chest (this is an in-breath) and together they create the gentle rocking motion through the body that is the signature of Free and Easy Wandering.

2. **Extended Arm Swing and Stride Pattern Walking:** Used when in a rush, or for a more targeted medical physical workout, but if sustained for too long it may induce excessive wear and tear on the knees, hips, pelvis and spine. It is best therefore to apply it in short bursts, where it will increase stamina and act as a tonic for both the cardiovascular and the respiratory systems.

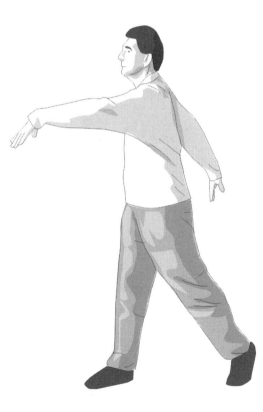

FIGURE 37: Extended Stride Walking

"He who strides cannot maintain the pace."
— *LAO-TSU*

3. **Middle Path Walking:** Generally considered to be a regular walking pace that gets us from A to B without rushing or delaying. It is nature's healthy walking pace and if performed correctly can create the impression of a body in perpetual motion.

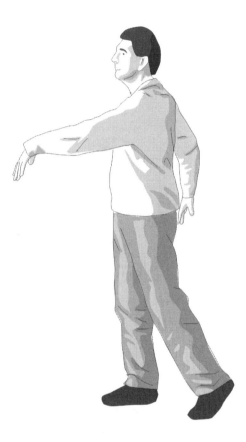

FIGURE 38 : Middle Path Walking

The Mechanics of Middle Path Walking

So here is the ultimate beginner's guide to regular Middle Path Walking. You are never too old to start learning it and, by doing so, you will gain instant benefits to your health and well-being. Let us examine the first step in Middle Path Walking, or Walking with the Dao:

- **The Head:** This is the home of three vital functions in the creation of natural walking: vision, intention and balance.

  Vision – Eyes should be placed on the distant horizon (halfway between heaven and earth). Do not floor-watch!

  Intention – This means "walking with purpose" and therefore it is important to match the intention to the chosen walking method. For example, you are in a rush to get from A to B, so you start Extended Stride Pattern Walking. This gets you there on time unless you have engaged the mind – the intention – of a Free and Easy Wanderer. If you have, you will get there relaxed but not on time. You should aim for a subtle combination of alertness, intention and calmness in order to arrive safe, on time and stress-free.

  Balance – the head should be held up from the crown, which levels the ears, which are the home of the main sensors of balance throughout the whole body.

- **The Chest:** This is the centre of gravity for the spine, which must be encouraged to flex forward and backward and twist sideways to propel the body forward.

- **The Shoulders:** These should be sliding over the upper ribcage, linking into the rhythmic muscular and joint-to-joint total body walking action.

- **The Arms:** Should be naturally falling away from the body with armpits open and swinging forwards and backwards – one open while the other closes. The action should resemble a pendulum swinging from the shoulder core, with the elbows leading both forward and backward swings. A forward-swung leading elbow opens the shoulder and a backward-swung leading elbow closes the shoulder.

- **The Pelvis:** This should tilt forward and back and twist left and right as the legs swing back and forth. It should act like a mid-body pumping station that flexes the spine and adds to the self-propulsion inherent in natural walking.

- **The Hips:** To remain loose, open and relaxed. A sense of "whole-leg swing" should be developed through the centre of the hips.

- **The Knees:** Also loose and relaxed, but you should encourage their natural springiness, because without this they will fail to propel you along and absorb the shock of when the leading heel makes contact with the ground.

- **The Feet:** It is vital to get these operating correctly: the leading foot should always make light contact with the earth through the heel as you spring off the ball and toes of the rear foot, using the springy tendons. When looking from the side, this manifests as a gentle bobbing up-and-down action. In addition, the feet should always be pointing forward; this centres and aligns the hips and knees for quality walking action and structural stability. The gap between the feet should be two to three inches, which drops the hip joint and allows it to swing naturally through its centre.

"About 10,000 *cases of breast and bowel cancer could be prevented in the UK if more people did more brisk walking."*
— *WORLD CANCER RESEARCH FUND SCIENTISTS*

- **Coiling in Walking:** You will notice when you walk that the arm swings forward to match the forward swing of the opposite leg. This happens for a good reason: to develop "Body Coiling" through the waist and torso, which makes the muscles move, coil and spring to propel you along. This coiling action drives the circulation throughout the whole body and opens and closes the chest cavity, making the lungs function more efficiently. This is the most important action of your body in health terms, because without coiling the body stagnates.

Walking with Spirit

- **Walking Through the Heart:** The heart is the home centre of the Shen (Spirit); to "stir the spirit" when walking you should focus on the chest centre to make your body feel light, vitalized and animated, lifting your mood and creating a feelgood factor.

  To walk through the heart, gently project yourself forward through the middle of the chest as you swing your leading leg forward.

- **Walking Through the Centre:** The main application of this is to "Direct and Project".

  It directs by pointing the way forward, left or right; the waist directs and the body follows. It projects by unconsciously moving of the gravity centre that pushes the Qi forward in the direction you are going.

  Note: The head directs the waist by instruction (internal subconscious guidance) and it leads it physically.

- **Sky Eye Walking:** This is practised by the Daoist elite, who are able to link their eyes and minds with the vibrations of the Dao externally, in the landscape that they are usually meandering through. They were able to "see" the presence of Qi in everything in a similar way some people claim to be able to "see" people's auras. Generally not open to mere mortals like you and me.

Health Benefits of Walking

Here are a number of health benefits that mechanically correct, natural Middle Path walking offers:

- A person of average build, walking for 30 minutes at 3.5 miles per hour, will burn off 140 calories. This is assuming you are walking at a regular pace on a reasonably flat surface, are engaging all the muscle groups and breathing deeply from the diaphragm.
- Walking enhances cardiovascular and pulmonary health (heart, breathing and general circulation). To maximise its efficiency it is advisable to start with a regular walking pace, then gradually increase it to Extended Stride pace, which should be maintained for a few minutes before returning to a regular pace again.
- Walking lowers cholesterol. The combination of increased cardiovascular activity and deeper abdominal/diaphragm breathing strengthens the metabolism and lowers cholesterol. High oxygen and low carbon levels keep the blood thin and less likely to clot.
- It strengthens the immune system by boosting white cell production. When walking, the force of gravity plus the moving weight of the body's soft tissues acting on the bones makes the brain fire up the production of white cells in the marrow.

- It helps lift mood and combats depression. It is not only the practice of walking that does this, but where you walk too; a beautiful scenic location helps.
- Studies show that regular walkers are less likely to develop the likes of Alzheimer's, diabetes and cancer. Stress is now being labelled the killer it was always suspected to be and it is no coincidence that regular walkers register low stress levels. All the above conditions are made worse by stress and are even thought to be more likely to develop in the first place.
- It builds stamina and fitness. It is a safe and gentle, low-impact way to build up general fitness levels. Start on a level flat surface and over a few weeks change the surface and increase the gradient. This will increase your lung capacity and boost the cardiovascular system.
- It keeps the brain sharp and oxygen-rich. The physical action of healthy walking opens the body to the extent that even the brain benefits: there is a significant increase in oxygen-rich red blood cells. You will notice your thinking is clearer, will feel energised and in good spirits.
- It helps counter the onset of osteoporosis. If you were to analyze the physical mechanics of walking you would find that the body tends to bob up and down. This is working directly on the bones of legs, pelvis and spine, which generates more cells for stronger bones.
- It helps fight arthritis and improves hip and knee function. Another reason why we should all walk in tune with gravity, in a light and open way that stimulates healthy circulation around all our joints.
- It helps the body retain its sense of balance. Healthy walking moves the body naturally and if practised regularly, the neuropathways that stem from the central nervous system are electrically stimulated. This strengthens and reinforces the information travelling between the brain and the body's proprioceptors that are essential sensors for our sense of balance.
- It is a great way to metabolise fat. An interesting fact is how hill walking burns off fatty cells: for example an average nine-stone woman walking up as little as a ten-degree gradient for one hour expends 590 calories. One reason for this is that walking on varied terrain engages and stimulates a broader range of muscles.

Walking with Parkinson's Disease

When I recently read a headline in a national newspaper: "Tai Chi can help Parkinson's patients to walk," I thought "Good, others are doing it as well." I have for some time been singing the praises of healthy walking mechanics and have applied this to a group with Parkinson's disease. My findings were that there was: general posture improvement; increased stride length; a reduction in upper-body stiffness; improved levels of energy and raised spirit; sense of well-being; and marked improvement in balance. I introduced Tai Chi walking to the group after I had first addressed their postural and muscular stiffness. Simply directing them to stand straight and walk correctly would not work with this disease unless I also worked on trying to rebalance their flexor muscles (psoas major and rectus abdominis among others) and extensor muscles (including the gluteus maximus and erector spinae), feet positioning and walking gait. I taught them how to bend, stretch and breathe in harmony and gradually adjusted their postures to a more open and balanced state. Then they walked, and the transformation happened.

It is also encouraging to hear of a study carried out by Dr Fuzhong Li and his team at the Oregon Research Institute in the USA. They suggest that Tai Chi could be used as an add-on to current physical therapies to address some of the key clinical problems in Parkinson's disease, such as postural and gait instability. The Parkinson's group I regularly teach is increasing in numbers because of the enhanced benefits they have experienced beyond the regular therapies they were offered; correctness of walking is a major part of this.

> *"Sometimes I'd walk, walk far from home,*
> *the things I've seen and I alone."*
> — *WANG WEI*, **Tang Dynasty**

Life is what you make it. To grow and experience life you have to be strong and healthy and prepared to seek it out. Wang Wei makes it clear that we should walk to "be strong" and to "see life", because neither will walk to us.

Questions and Answers

When I walk up any incline I soon become breathless. What do you think is the cause?

I assume you have had problems with your cardiovascular and pulmonary systems ruled out by your doctor, because both of these could cause breathlessness. Otherwise it could be posture/circulation related, maybe "Fixed Excessive" posture. This is when the spine operates in constant extension (bowed inwards, chest out), or flexion (bowed outwards, chest in). Either of these will throw your breathing and walking mechanics out. Constriction of the blood vessels starves the muscles and brain of essential oxygen and thus can have an impact on energy levels and breathing. The posture problem can be rectified with the guidance in this book, but any problems involving pain in the legs, head or chest when walking should be reported to your doctor immediately.

How often and how far should I walk?

You should practise all three methods of walking described in this chapter every day to maximize their health benefits. The distance you cover should be middling (not too much and not too little).

After only ten minutes of Extended Stride Pattern walking, I notice my lower back starts to feel tight. What am I doing wrong?

I think you are doing it for too long a period. Extended Stride Pattern should only be applied in short bursts – five minutes at a time. Additionally, you could be putting too much power into the forward driving of the body, which is overextending your spine (pushing your chest out too far) and creating excessive inward curvature of your lumbar joints. Another reason for backache could be that you are landing too heavily on your heel, which creates a powerful upward rebounding force that can stiffen the muscles of the lumbar spine.

I am a classic Toes Splayed walker and suffer hip and knee pain. How can I rectify this?

A quick and easy answer is to bring your feet back in line and realign the hips and knees. But I know it's not as simple as that, so here are some ideas for you to try:

1. Become "Feet Conscious"; every time you walk or just stand, look down and make a spot check on where they are pointing.

2. Be patient and allow time for your feet to adjust. It can take weeks or even months for the supporting soft tissues of the knees, hips and pelvis to return to their home centre.

3. To make the physical adjustments to the ankles and/or feet, there are two ways to gently ease and encourage the tissues to realign with gravity.

Firstly, stand with your feet shoulder-width apart (place your hands on a tabletop or worktop for stability) and lift the heels slightly off the ground. Then pivot on the balls of the feet, ease the heels in towards each other and lower the heels. Hold for ten seconds. Then repeat but this time with the heels opening out away from each other and lower the heels down. Hold for twenty seconds and repeat the whole process three more times. This stimulates calf, shin and thigh muscles to adapt to the required new shape.

Secondly, resume the same stance, only this time bring the weight into the heels and lift the toes off the ground. Pivot on the heels to swivel the toes out, then lower them down and hold for ten seconds. Repeat but with the toes turning in, lower down and hold for twenty seconds.

Note of caution: Do not twist the feet in or out forcefully; reach the point where you feel a slight resistance and hold at that position. Not to be attempted if you have arthritis, osteoporosis or any other bone and muscular conditions.

How will Tai Chi Walking help my sciatic pain?

Irrespective of what is the root cause of your sciatica, correct walking mechanics will definitely be of help to release the pressure on the sciatic nerve. Tightness across the sacrum and out to the hips can be one major cause of sciatica and is due to the hidden deep muscle called the piriformis. This band of muscle connects to the sacrum and femur head and is prone to pressing down on the sciatic nerve that passes directly under it. Normally when the sacrum and hip are open, flexing and healthy it remains above the nerve with no contact, but when stiffness affects the sacrum and the hip that it connects to, it too can stiffen and weaken, causing it to drop down onto the sciatic nerve, which can be extremely painful.

An effective way to free the hips and sacrum is to place a book on the floor. Place one foot on it and stand up straight. The other leg/hip will now be hanging in mid-air. Steady yourself by placing one hand on the wall and commence swinging the free leg as if walking at a regular pace. Do this twelve times on each leg. This releases the hip and sacrum on that side of the body and loosens the piriformis.

Now repeat on the other leg for hip and pelvic balance. Finish off by removing the book and standing in Upright Squat (see Figure 30, page 119). While in this posture, gently bounce up and down, shaking the hips and pelvic girdle. Then swivel the waist left and right a bit like the "Chubby Checker" explained earlier. Twist while bending and straightening the knees. This usually does the trick.

8

The "Stillness" of Self-Healing – The Untapped Source for Healing

Stillness makes me happy
Stillness makes me smile,
In stillness I find all I need,
So here I'll stay a while.

— *PTN*

According to the ancient Tai Chi masters stillness is a vital ingredient in the search for enlightenment; so in this chapter, we will explore its meaning, how it can be found, utilized and sustained to contribute to healing power. In order to create an atmosphere of understanding the essence of stillness, I have loaded this chapter with poetic verse, which in my opinion is the best way to transmit its message.

"When the body is at rest (sitting or standing), it should be as still as a mountain."
— *CLASSICS OF WANG CHUNG-YUEH*

Meaning

What is stillness in the context of the Dao? It is a real force, a stabilizing force that is the glue of the universe and permeates all matter. It is Yin in its most pure form and according to the Daoist writer John Blofeld (known as the Ox-Head Recluse): "No concepts! No thought at all! Stillness, perfect stillness!" There are two distinct ways to look at stillness:

1. **Stillness Within** – The way to understand stillness within is to imagine the deep stillness of night, which envelops everything, creating the impression that everything is still. Yet within the darkness rivers still flow, trees still bend with the wind that still blows and the night's creatures still patrol their territory. So within the apparent stillness, the cycle of life continues. This is the stillness that should be experienced within.

> *An empty mind*
> *No thoughts distract,*
> *My spirit calm and centred.*
> *For here I sit where three*
> *Are one, the realm of*
> *"Stillness" entered.*
> — *P T N*

A centred body creates a centred mind. A centred body and mind creates a centred spirit – now all three are one in stillness.

2. **Stillness Without** – Is the external projection of the stillness within, the ambience of a peaceful exterior and a visible contented spirit. It also encompasses the stillness found in nature, most notably in the mountains, which is where the Daoist recluses retreated, to find not only themselves, but also the Dao.

> *Stillness Mountain*
> *To Stillness Mountain they came,*
> *The young, the old, the poor, the lame.*
> *Despite the cost, despite the pain,*
> *To Stillness Mountain they came.*
>
> *And what was it that they sought?*
> *A gold-filled mine, an emperor's court?*
> *What they desired could not be bought*
> *And stillness was its name.*
>
> *They came to find the truth, but*
> *Found a sage instead,*
> *Who taught them nothing about nothing*
> *And nothing is what he said.*

Their steps now light, their steps now
Few, lie gently on the mountain dew
And whispers on the wind that blew,
Cries "Stillness is their home".

— *P T N*

In the context of the Tai Chi symbol, stillness is found in five locations:

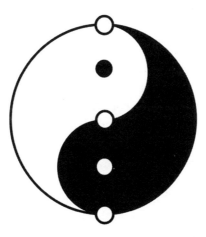

FIGURE 39: Five Points of Stillness

1. At the absolute core centre of the whole symbol. This is the gravitational core of the spiralling energy that is Tai Chi. It is the calm
   eye at the centre of the storm, the inactive within the active, the
   stillness within stillness and the stillness within motion. This is the
   centre – the point of balance that gives us the much sought-after
   Central Equilibrium.
   EXAMPLE IN PRACTICE: Recently, a student of mine to whom
   I had given advice on how to find his true centre in life walked
   into my class and thanked me for clearing his eczema from his
   hands. He said since he reorganized his life, his perspectives and
   his personal health training, a sense of calm had appeared and his
   eczema dissolved away. I had seen his hands earlier and knew his
   acute eczema was being fed by his stressful life. His hands were now
   clear and smooth. He had found his centre.

2. At the point of Yang to Yin transition at the top of the symbol. When energy rises (Yang) there will come a point where its force will be spent and for just a few short seconds stillness appears, before it falls back to earth drawn by the force of gravity (Yin). You can see this in the weightless training undergone by astronauts, which achieves its state of stillness (weightlessness) at the point where the plane levels off after its steep climb.
    EXAMPLE IN PRACTICE: It is the point your body takes you to at the absolute top of a natural morning stretch, when you wake up from the stillness of sleep.

3. At the point of Yin to Yang transition at the bottom of the symbol. This is where the force of Yin transforms into Yang and just at the point of transfer stillness is experienced.
    EXAMPLE IN PRACTICE: This is where the body "falls" to at the deepest point in the sleeping cycle and the transition moment as we begin to surface from our slumbers.

4. At the heart of the rising Yang lies the stillness of Yin, the anchor of active Yang Qi. Without this stabilizer, Yang Qi would become unstable, rampant and destructive.
    EXAMPLE IN PRACTICE: In ancient China, the greatest warriors would demonstrate a calmness on the chaotic battlefield that defied logic. This was however the reason why they would survive – they retained a clearness of mind when all the others around them had lost theirs.

5. At the heart of the descending Yin lies the opposing uplifting force of Yang, the "Ridgepole" that gives Yin Qi form and without which Yin would lose its creative harmony with Yang and disperse. While Yin descends in its fullness of power, Yang holds firm to stabilize in stillness and strength.
    EXAMPLE IN PRACTICE: A parachutist leaps from a plane and is falling to earth – to those witnessing the event on the ground, at an alarming rate. However, from the parachutist's perspective the experience is different; he or she is quite relaxed but alert, calm yet excited as he or she sits in stillness at the heart of the plummeting force of Yin.

Sung and Fang Sung

The Sung of Stillness
Stillness is my source of light,
Stillness makes me strong.
Stillness where my true self lies,
In stillness, I find Sung.

Sung is where my body rests,
Relaxes and feels free.
Sung lies quiet within our hearts,
Where she waits for you and me.

If stillness guides us to our Sung
And Sung leads us to the Dao,
Then the Dao is home to both
And she's waiting for us now.
— PTN

Sung's literal translation is "To Relax", but there is no limit to its meaning. Sung can mean to physically relax the whole body, relax the mind, relax the Jinglo (Energy Body) and even feel your Shen (Living Spirit) relax.

I move, I breathe, I feel, I see,
My spirit raised so naturally
And now the calm envelops me,
I've found the Dao through Sung.
— PTN

Fang Sung means to "Relax, Let Go and Release", but I would add something else: Relax, Let Go, Release and Receive. In short, this is Sung but with an extra dimension, where *you* the Living Spirit commune with the universal Qi that surrounds our bodies – this is pure stillness. The goal is to achieve Quan Shen Fang Sung, which translates to "Whole Body Relaxed".

Fang Sung is a content and peaceful heart
And a temple for a radiant spirit.
— PTN

153

You can read about my "big impact" experience with Sung in my first book *The Middle Path of Tai Chi*. Here I would like to share with you an equally astounding first encounter with Fang Sung that one can only describe as enlightening.

Fang Sung Transparency

Internal Classic number 10 is titled "Seek Serenity in Activity", which is exactly what I experienced during an early morning workout in a valley in beautiful Wales. There is a saying in the world of Tai Chi that describes what I experienced for the first time that morning: "Soaring on the winds of Qi". I had arrived at the exercise spot just after 6.00 am; this is a valley that 200 years ago had a tributary of the river Conwy running through it. I set about my usual routines of Qigong exercises followed by a Tai Chi choreographed form.

The valley also lies at the end of the Conwy valley, which is fed from the Snowdonia mountain range. Instead of facing the rising sun located at the foot of the valley as I usually would do, I decided on this morning to face up the valley into a warm breeze that originated high on the slopes of Mount Snowdon. This day felt different; the temperature was comfortably warm as you would expect in May and the air quality was as usual crisp and fresh, but there was something else.

I became aware of a tingling heaviness in the atmosphere all around me, which I assumed must be the Earth Qi my Chinese teachers had told me about. I think what followed was possible only because I had already reached a state of Sung by then. For some unknown reason I started to perform a standing exercise with fixed feet, a moving meditative internal exercise Master Chu King Hung calls Heaven and Earth Qigong (see Chapter 5). Within seconds I felt as if my whole body had been lifted off the ground by an unseen force. It was like skydiving standing upright; I had become a kite in the wind, which seemed not only to elevate me but to blow straight through me as well. My body felt transparent and my breathing enveloped it, creating a sensation of soaring. All thoughts had dissolved into this one moment and for the first time in my life I felt that I had "Let Go".

I had just experienced Fang Sung and since that time I have been able to find it at will, as if I had stepped through a door into a realm that had previously been closed to me. Embracing Fang Sung offers you a simple way to find inner peace in a pressurised world.

"When inordinate desire is banished, no errant thoughts arise. The mind is stilled; the spirit becomes radiant and its brilliance illumines all the mysteries of the universe. then there is no limit to the marvellous powers attained."
— *CHOU SHAO-HSIEN*

Twenty years ago when I set up the China Bridge Tai Chi and Qigong School, I scoured the ancient proverbs for a school motto and found the above. We can all benefit from its simple but enlightening message:

"When inordinate desire is banished" – Craving is a destructive negative force generated by a weak human mind.

"No errant thoughts arise" – Craving tilts the emotions out of balance, which dislodges the centred wisdom mind that normally controls the feral children that are the emotions. When emotions rule errant thoughts are free to arise.

"The mind is stilled" – By banishing the inordinate desire of excessive craving, the Monkey Mind quietens and stillness appears out of nowhere.

"The spirit becomes radiant" – If you sustain the state of stillness for long enough, the usually tainted Spirit (Shen) will become radiant, fed from the increased levels of subtle Qi that have built up in a now healthier body and mind. A radiant Spirit is on the earthly plane, experienced as feeling robust in health and energy, with a contented and positive mind.

"Its brilliance illumines all the mysteries of the universe" – When the spirit is nurtured through the meditative practice of stillness, it is able to transcend to what the ancients called Cosmic Qi. This is when your earthbound spirit raises its frequency to much higher levels and the door to immortality opens.

"Then there is no limit to the marvellous powers attained" – To live for ever, to travel through time and space and to understand the great Dao: all these things are what the ancient Daoist masters called "Achievable by the few."

Be still my sky, be still my earth
And all that dwells between.

— *P T N*

Questions and Answers

What is meditation and what has stillness to do with this?
Meditation is the method adopted by the ancient Buddhist and Daoist adepts to find inner peace, stillness and enlightenment. A simplified explanation: the word "meditation" breaks down to "medi" = centre or middle; therefore this is the practice that guides us to the middle. It is the middle where we will find peace, balance and stillness.

The Dove
The dove sits in silent repose
Lost in uncomplicated thoughts.
— *P T N*

What is the difference between stillness and to be still?
This depends on whether it is viewed from a Western or an Eastern perspective:

Western: both mean the same – something that is not moving.

Eastern: stillness has depth, profundity and mystery. To be still does not mean simply not moving.

I will never be able to be as still as you suggest. So why should I bother?
Stillness is relative to each individual. The stillness of a sage is incomprehensible to a complete novice; it all depends on your character (Teh) as to how deeply you can immerse yourself. A little is better than none.

When I try to be still my mind won't slow down. How do I do this?
This is also down to character, plus how life has influenced you. The most important virtue in this scenario is patience. A mind that won't switch off is called a Monkey Mind. In order to calm the monkey it must be starved and not fed. This is achieved by doing nothing, because doing something means you are engaging the brain, which fires up the monkey-driven electric circuitry you are desperate to switch off.

Many of us are external in mind; this means that focusing inward in meditative practice does not come easily, making it more difficult to connect to our minds. This difficulty and the ever-working mind are fed by the pressures of modern life. Meditation is of course mainly associated with Eastern cultures and practices, but with guidance, patience and practice we can all work on our Monkey Minds.

> EXAMPLE IN PRACTICE: Sit still in a quiet spot and do nothing but breathe; after only a few minutes you will notice the monkey calming down.

I suffer from regular bouts of migraine; could stillness be a useful way to combat this?
Stillness on its own will help you stay calm, which lessens the potential for migraine and will help you recover more quickly during one. But if you can learn to incorporate the all-powerful stillness in moving exercise, you will broaden its healing potential. You can try walking, bending, stretching, twisting and running – lightly on the balls of the feet, not heel-jogging on hard surfaces.

9

The Science –
Research into Tai Chi
and Qigong

Let knowledge and nature
Lead us to the pathway home.
— *P T N*

During the last thirty years there have been many research studies carried out on the health benefits of Tai Chi and Qigong. I have collected some together here.

Cardiovascular

"In our study, pulse measurements showed that Tai Chi specifically improved expansion and contraction of the arteries, known as arterial compliance."
— *DR WILLIAM TSANG,*
Hong Kong Polytechnic University

This is down to two things. First, the way Tai Chi relaxes not only the surface muscles but also the deep muscle fibres to create what is known as an "Empty Body". This is when the heart is free from the "Back Pressure" of a tense body that forms resistance to its natural pumping action. Secondly, the way the whole body when practising Tai Chi moves in a snake-like pulsing, rhythmic and integrated manner, which the Chinese call "Chan Su Jin" (Silk Reeling Energy). In tandem with the breathing, this stimulates all the body's blood vessels to stretch, flex, expand and contract, keeping them pliable and healthy, thus creating the results quoted in the research.

Osteoporosis

"Over a nine-month period, we studied two groups of women with osteoporosis: one undertook Tai Chi, the other standard weight-based training. The Tai Chi group gained 0.5% bone density over the period while the other lost 1%."

— **DR PETER WAYNE,**

Harvard Medical School, USA

"When we put weight down through the long bones, by adding Tai Chi's spiral force the muscles attached to them pull against the periosteum (the outer covering layer of the bones). When this force is applied to the periosteum, the brain sends signals to the body to make more calcium and deposits it in the bone tissue to strengthen them against the force being applied. When the out-breath is added to this exercise, the weight load and stretch against the bone reaches its maximum loading. This is why this kind of spiral exercise, where the muscle is worked through its full range, is so good at strengthening long bones on a regular basis against the natural effects of ageing."

— **SUSI SHEEN,**

Chartered Physiotherapist

Mental Illness/Stress

"A study was carried out to evaluate the effects of Tai Chi and Qigong practice on individuals with traumatic brain injury. Twenty individuals practised for an hour a week over the course of eight weeks and then answered a questionnaire to measure mood, self-esteem and flexibility among other aspects. Early findings showed an improvement in mood and self-esteem."

— **THE FACULTY OF MEDICINE AND HEALTH SCIENCES,**

University of Nottingham, UK

"According to a medical study undertaken by psychiatrists at the University of California, adding a mind-body exercise programme to older adult's treatments improved their outcomes in the treatment of depression."

— **Results to be published in the Journal of Geriatric Psychiatry**

"Tai Chi's precise movements relieve depression, boost self-esteem and reduce stress and anxiety."
— *DR CHENCHEN WANG*, Tufts University School
of Medicine, Massachusetts, USA

The opening and closing body movements of Tai Chi and Qigong increase oxygen supply to the brain cells. This helps clear a cloudy melancholy mind by energizing the cells and making the individual more mentally alert. It is also worth noting that the pulsing wave-like movements of Tai Chi's choreographed patterns create a rocking motion that is known to release endorphins in the brain, making us feel more relaxed and calm.

Additionally, the Tai Chi postures are a stimulus for the Shen (Spirit), which creates mental (and physical) strength. Recent studies have shown that Tai Chi increases the level of serotonin in the blood; low levels of serotonin are linked with depression and higher levels with better mood.

Prevention of Falls

"Elderly people who regularly practised Tai Chi not only showed better proprioception at the ankle and knee joints than sedentary controls, but also better ankle kinesthesis than swimmers/runners. The large benefits of Tai Chi exercise on proprioception may result in the maintenance of balance control in older people."
— *PROFESSOR Y HONG*, Department of Sports Science and Physical
Education, the Chinese University of Hong Kong

"The performance of the choreographed Tai Chi form over a half-hour period uses up the same amount of energy as brisk walking. When comparing the overall benefits of Tai Chi form versus brisk walking in a group of previously sedentary seventy-year-olds, the Tai Chi group did better on several counts, with stronger lower limb muscles, greater flexibility and improved balance."
— *JOSEPH AUDETTE*, Professor of Rehabilitation, Harvard Medical School

"Elderly people whose eyesight is failing can improve their balance and avoid falls by practising Tai Chi."
— *DR WILLIAM TSANG*, Hong Kong Polytechnic University

I read a recent report from S.L.Wolf and colleagues, from the Atlanta FICSIT Group, that to me is quite profound. They say "Tai Chi exercise reduces the risk of falling by 47.5%." Can you imagine the cost saving to our nation's health budgets if Tai Chi was promoted and made available to all over-fifties?

A healthily functioning proprioception system is essential in reducing the likelihood of falls happening. This is the body's neurological biofeedback system and keeps your brain constantly informed of the body's balance, both in stillness and in motion. Falls are known to occur when this system degrades through factors including lack of stimulation, natural ageing and external complications like: brain injury, chemotherapy and inner ear conditions. The perfect coordination of the joints and muscles in Tai Chi and Qigong stimulates the body's Energy Meridian System to become more conductive, which clears the neuropathways to send and receive messages.

Cancer Treatment and Prevention

"In a study of Qigong therapy on breast cancer patients treated with chemotherapy, the twenty-one-day programme showed a significant difference in white blood cells, platelets and haemoglobin, suggesting that Qigong therapy may decrease leukopenia in breast cancer patients treated with chemo."
— **Cancer Nursing Journal 29**

"Recent research shows regular exercising reduces the risk of breast cancer recurring by 40%, of prostate cancer by 30% and of bowel cancer by 5%."
— *PROFESSOR ROBERT THOMAS*, **Bedford and Cambridge University Hospitals, UK**

Ciaran Devan, Chief Executive of Macmillan Cancer Support, recently said:

"Cancer patients would be shocked if they knew how much of a benefit physical activity could have on their recovery and long-term health."

If someone decided to search for the perfect exercise therapy for cancer sufferers, the experts would do well to save themselves a lot of time and effort by proposing Tai Chi and Qigong. Below I list all the areas of concern you would want this sophisticated exercise system to cover and assess the viability of Tai Chi and

Qigong as the solution:

CANCER SIDE EFFECTS	TAI CHI AND QIGONG OPTIONS
Anxiety:	Tai Chi is proven to lift the mood by raising serotonin levels
Tiredness and Fatigue:	Naturally raises energy levels by making the body more oxygen-rich
Compromised Immunity:	Boosts the immune system
Lymphoedema:	The breathing, muscular stimulation, body-mechanics and postures move lymph fluid
Chemo Cloudy Brain:	Oxygen levels increase in the brain, clearing the thinking
Pain, general or localized:	The exercises move pain by moving Qi to disperse Tui Na massage (discussed later on) also moves pain
Nerve Damage to Hands/Feet:	Qi is directed to the hands and feet to speed up recovery
Constipation and Diarrhoea:	Tui Na circular massage of the large intestine

Diabetes

In recent research, a twelve-week programme of Tai Chi led to a significant fall of 8 per cent in blood sugar levels in those suffering Type 2 diabetes, which is linked to obesity. The exercises also boosted the body's immune system. This is significant because an improved immune system damps down the chronic in-flammation of the body's internal organs associated with diabetes.

In another study, a twelve-week programme of Tai Chi and Qigong resulted in a significant fall in blood glucose levels. Insulin resistance also improved significantly. The complete package of exercises, breathing training and massage is ideal for diabetes sufferers, as indicated in the above research. Not mentioned, though, is the further benefit of how Tai Chi and Qigong open up the fine capillaries of the body, especially in the extremities (hands and feet). The postures and the pulsing, rhythmic exercises associated with Tai Chi and Qigong are perfect for the complications that may arise out of diabetes. Organs can breathe and major blood vessels and all the fine capillaries dilate to increase the healing blood flow to all the tissues of the body.

Stroke

"Practising a Tai Chi short form improves balance for stroke sufferers in a twelve-week study of 136 subjects who had one hour's tuition a week followed by a further three hours a week self-practice."

— **The Department of Rehabilitation Services, Hong Kong Polytechnic University**

The balance of these patients improved through the Tai Chi principle of Mind – Intention – Completion:

1. The mind is activated by the initial thought of what they wish to accomplish.

2. The next step is their intention to move the body, which creates EMF (electro-motive force).

3. Finally, we have completion, which is when the EMF has expressed itself through the body to the end of the movement.

When we practise Tai Chi Form (a series of connected choreographed moving postures), we are encouraged to look where we want to move to, visualize the movement, then execute it. All this is collectively linked to the subtle ebb and flow of the Qi breath. This method, unique to Tai Chi, is called "Leading with the Qi". This means the mind + intention = spirit-driven movement, which sends Qi down the limbs just before they actually move; and where Qi flows, the blood follows. I use this method often in my remedial therapy work and have had some success in improving limb sensation and movement.

Immune System

"A five-month study was carried out to ascertain whether the practice of Tai Chi could improve the immune response to the flu vaccine in older adults. They found a significant increase in the size and duration of the antibody response in the control group of Tai Chi practitioners."
— **The University of Illinois, USA**

The lymphatic system relies on muscular expansions and contractions and gravitational drainage to pump the lymphatic fluid around the body, which is why Tai Chi is perfect for this function. This fluid needs to move to cleanse the body of toxic nasties; plus, the angles we lift the arms up to (above the shoulder line) and the shapes the torso makes in conjunction are helpful for natural lymph drainage.

Parkinson's Disease

"A comparative study of fifty-six Parkinson's sufferers who undertook ninety minutes of Qigong training (compared to a group not practising Qigong) a week over the course of a year showed significant improvement to the disruptive motor symptoms in Parkinson's disease."
— **The University of Bonn, Germany**

"According to recent research a brisk walk could improve the symptoms of Parkinson's. The study of sixty people with mild to moderate Parkinson's who were asked to walk briskly three times a week showed improvements of between 7 and 15% across the following areas: motor function, mood, fatigue, general fitness and thinking abilities."
— *DR ERGUN UC.,* **University of Iowa Craver College of Medicine, USA**

Now this report may not on the face of it sound ground-breaking, but to the many people who are suffering this debilitating disease it certainly is. Just ask the group I teach in the UK (who are consistently growing in number) what impact Tai Chi has had on the quality of their lives.

The disruptive motor symptoms referred to here are caused by the blocking of the electrical impulses (Qi) that flow between the body and the brain. These include loss of focus and concentration (cloudy brain), impairment to speech, weakening of the structural muscles causing slumped posture, stiffness of the muscles, tremors, cramps, spasms and high probability of falls.

This list of symptoms is what I actually see and experience with my Parkinson's students, and although they may sound dire, practising Tai Chi and Qigong offers Parkinson's sufferers real relief with no nasty side effects. The secret to the effectiveness of these arts lies in the way they influence all the internal functions of the human body and in the words of the doctors of Traditional Chinese Medicine: "Tai Chi and Qigong removes 'Sickly Qi' (blocked and stagnant energy, which if left unchecked will cause damage to all human cells), which causes stagnation and blockage in the body." When you consider all that you will appreciate why the organisations that represent Parkinson's sufferers throughout the world are finally taking notice of this amazing healing art. For more details on the impact of Tai Chi Walking for Parkinson's, see Chapter 7, Health Benefits.

Arthritis

"Regular exercise is vital to keep your joints healthy and long-term benefits of exercise far outweigh the risk of injury."
— *PROFESSOR MARK BATT*, consultant in sport and exercise medicine, Nottingham University Hospitals, UK

"Research has shown that the body's joints, bones and cartilage rely on the stimulation of physical activity to repair themselves. If you don't use the affected joint it will get worse."
— *PROFESSOR ALAN SILMAN*, Medical Director, Arthritis Research UK

I particularly like the report from researchers at the Daejeon University, Korea who carried out a twelve-week study with a group of rheumatoid arthritis sufferers. After practising for only fifty minutes a week there was a significant decrease in pain and fatigue. In the past rheumatoid arthritis sufferers were reluctant to exercise because it just seemed to inflame the condition more. But that was based on typical Western physical exercising, which is more muscle-focused in its methods. Tai Chi and Qigong is much softer and lower-impact on sensitive joints and is now proving to work on this condition.

In the not too distant past the advice given by well-meaning health professionals to arthritis sufferers (especially rheumatoid) was to "rest". This, according to Professor Silman, "was clearly the wrong advice". He suggests "The right exercise at the right time is hugely beneficial and the worst thing people can do is to do nothing." The right exercise is Tai Chi and Qigong and the right time is NOW! In the UK more than 10 million people suffer from arthritis and in the

USA over 52 million are afflicted by this disabling condition. The numbers speak for themselves and are a damning indictment of our lifestyles. We need for a start to stop consuming high-sugar food and drinks, as researchers have found that as soon as glucose is ingested by the body, it has an inflammatory effect on the joints. I am not a scientist or a dietician, but what I do know is that the spiralling, wave-like pulsing actions of Tai Chi and Qigong open and close the joints, which has a cleansing effect, washing out the damaging inflammatory toxins.

Note: Just moving the joints sometimes or slightly is not enough; you have to move all your joints daily through their full range of movement and Tai Chi and Qigong are uniquely placed to do just that.

Pulmonary Conditions

Asthma

"After a six-week programme for seventeen adult patients to perform Tai Chi exercises at home on a daily basis, there were significant improvements to: peak flow variability (with a rise in oxygen consumption level,) control of asthma and quality of life."

— **Department of Medicine, Ramathibodi Hospital, Thailand**

I was not surprised by the results of this research, specifically because I had worked with a large group of children with asthma in the 1990s. After only a few weeks word of this had reached the BBC, who sent a reporter and film crew to interview the children and myself. They reported that everyone who attended the class noticed an improvement in the quality of their breathing and it appeared the children were having fewer episodes.

COPD (Chronic Obstructive Pulmonary Disease)

"From a total of forty-two patients with COPD and an average age of seventy-three, half undertook a twelve-week program of Tai Chi, while the other half received standard rehab. The Tai Chi group trained thirty minutes a day and at the end of the study they outperformed the other group in: improved balance; lower levels of depression and anxiety; stronger muscle strength in lower limbs; and extended duration of walking and increased speed of walking. Generally the Tai Chi group 'felt' better than the non-Tai Chi group."

— *REGINA WAN MAN LEUNG*, **Concord Repatriation General Hospital and the University of Sydney, Australia**

Just one look at the results of this research should be enough to tell anyone that Tai Chi can enhance and support all aspects of our lives. In just twelve weeks balance, depression, anxiety, muscle strength, breathing and quality of walking were all impacted upon by nature's administrator. What is not reported here is that the group would undoubtedly also have noticed all of their senses and bodily functions showing a marked improvement.

Multiple Sclerosis

"There was a pilot study of eight individuals who suffer from MS covering a two-month period. Statistically the pilot study found an intervention of six sessions of individual Tai Chi and Qigong instruction supplemented by audio and video teaching aids produced significant improvements in depression and balance across the group as a whole. Specific improvements were also reported on a range of other symptoms including spasms, numbness, bladder control and walking."

— **Research group headed by** *NICK MILLS BSC, MPHIL, C. PSYCHOL.* **(consultant clinical psychologist and qigong practitioner), Gwent Healthcare NHS Trust and Tai Chi Rehab, UK**

This study, although small in scale, threw up results that are worth noting and following up on, hopefully with a much larger sample. From my own experience working with people who are living with MS, I can concur with the above findings. With a little guidance from a Tai Chi and Qigong remedial therapist, MS sufferers are encouraged to direct Qi into limbs that may have lain dormant for some time, which helps fire up the motorization again (albeit usually in a limited way). I have also observed their mood and optimism improving when they are experiencing what to them is a significant change. One exercise I do with people living with MS is to teach them to apply Chinese Tui Na massage to their limbs in the form of gentle slapping, squeezing and rubbing of the muscles). Then I show them how to move their arms and legs using the correct extension and recoiling method.

Alzheimer's Disease

"Exercising three times a week for twenty minutes a time will reduce the risk of developing Alzheimer's Disease."

— *PROFESSOR CAROL BRAYNE.* **Cambridge University, UK**

This study found that regular exercise could cut the potential for developing Alzheimer's – "even just by walking to work". The combination of Healthy Living and Tai Chi Walking would fit perfectly into the exercise regime we should all adopt to help ward off this serious disease. The brain needs a constant oxygen-enriched blood supply and I cannot think of any other discipline that would achieve this better than Tai Chi and Qigong.

Summary

In all my years of involvement in these arts I have never seen such interest being shown in them by the Western medical fraternity. There must be huge sums of money being allocated for research and the pleasing thing is the majority of findings are positive. This last chapter I think reflects this and I hope offers some comfort to those who suffer from the conditions highlighted. Western medicine is vital in the fight against these debilitating illnesses and I am constantly heartened when hearing of a new breakthrough in the treatment of them. I think there is still a lot to learn not just from Chinese medicine and health practices, but from all corners of the world. It is my fervent hope that we will discover cures for the likes of cancer, Parkinson's, Alzheimer's and MS and that these cures will come from both the cutting-edge minds of our modern-day scientists and the remedies of our ancient cultures.

Regarding the book in general, I hope this will be one of the self-help guides you reach for first when you need advice on how to overcome or cope with your health issues.

On a personal level, I intend the book to become my main teaching reference manual for the rest of my teaching life. You see, we Tai Chi and Qigong teachers never retire… we just "Slow Down".

Acknowledgements

I would like to thank the following people who have either directly or indirectly assisted or inspired me to write this book:

LESLEY NEWTON – For her patience, love and support.

RICHARD NEWTON – For his truth and love.

JANINE SESSIONS – For her love and encouragement.

JEFF CUSHING – For his superb illustrations and observations.

CAROLYN RIDDING – For her belief and support.

IAN BEGBIE – For his humour, his wisdom and his vision.

MASTER YANG JWING-MING – For his foreword and for being a guiding light on the science of the human body.

MASTER MICHAEL TSE – For his excellent Qigong and making me realize the potential.

MASTER CHU KING HUNG – For opening my eyes to the power of Tai Chi.

JOYCE ROBERTS – Just for being my mum.

SABINE, CAROL & THIERRY – For seeing the potential.

ALL THE STUDENTS of China Bridge Tai Chi – For seeing what we see.

Bibliography

BLOFELD, JOHN. *Taoism: the Quest for Immortality* (Mandala Unwin Hyman Limited, 1989).

CLEARY, THOMAS. *Vitality, Energy, Spirit: A Taoist Sourcebook* (Shambhala Publications, Inc., 1991).

JOHNSON, JERRY ALAN. *Chinese Medical Qigong Therapy* (The International Institute of Medical Qigong, 2000).

LEGGE, JAMES. *The I Ching* (Dover Publications, Inc., 1963).

WINDRIDGE, CHARLES. *Tong Sing: the Chinese Book of Wisdom* (Kyle Cathie Limited, 2002).

WONG, EVA. *Cultivating Stillness* (Shambhala Publications Inc., 1992).

ZHANG MINGWU, SUN XINGYUAN. *Chinese Qigong Therapy* (Shandong Science and Technology Press, 1985).

About the Author

Sifu Peter Newton is married with two children (adults) and lives in Wales, UK. He is a full-time professional registered Tai Chi and Qigong teacher (Sifu) and works as a physical therapist. In 2009, he was invited to become an Honorary Vice-President of the 'Tai Chi Union for Great Britain' and for the last twenty years has specialized in and researched into the health enhancing benefits of Tai Chi and Qigong. His skills derive mainly from the training he has undertaken with three famous Tai Chi Grandmasters (Chu King-Hung, Michael Tse and Dr Yang Jwing-Ming); Dr Yang has kindly contributed the foreword to the book.

The physical therapy Peter practises is uniquely based on the body-mechanics of Tai Chi and Qigong and has attracted the attention of international footballers, the medical-care profession and the business world. For more information please visit his website: *www.chinabridgetaichi.co.uk*

Index

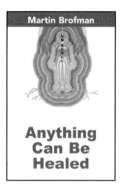

MARTIN BROFMAN

Anything Can Be Healed

This healer's tutorial and reference book looks at the physical body as a mirror of the consciousness within, with specific tensions on the physical level being reflected in the mind.

ISBN: 9781844090167

MEGAN CARNARIUS

A Deeper Perspective on Alzheimer's
and other Dementias

A compassionate, professional look at dementia, offering invaluable practical insights into care as well as into the spiritual dimensions of the disease.

ISBN: 9781844096626

FINDHORN PRESS

Life-Changing Books

Consult our catalogue online
(with secure order facility) on
www.findhornpress.com

For information on the Findhorn Foundation:
www.findhorn.org